Dash Diet Cookbook for Beginners

– Fight Against Hypertension and Coronary Artery Diseases with Healthy and Low Sodium Recipes –

[Sebastian Osborne]

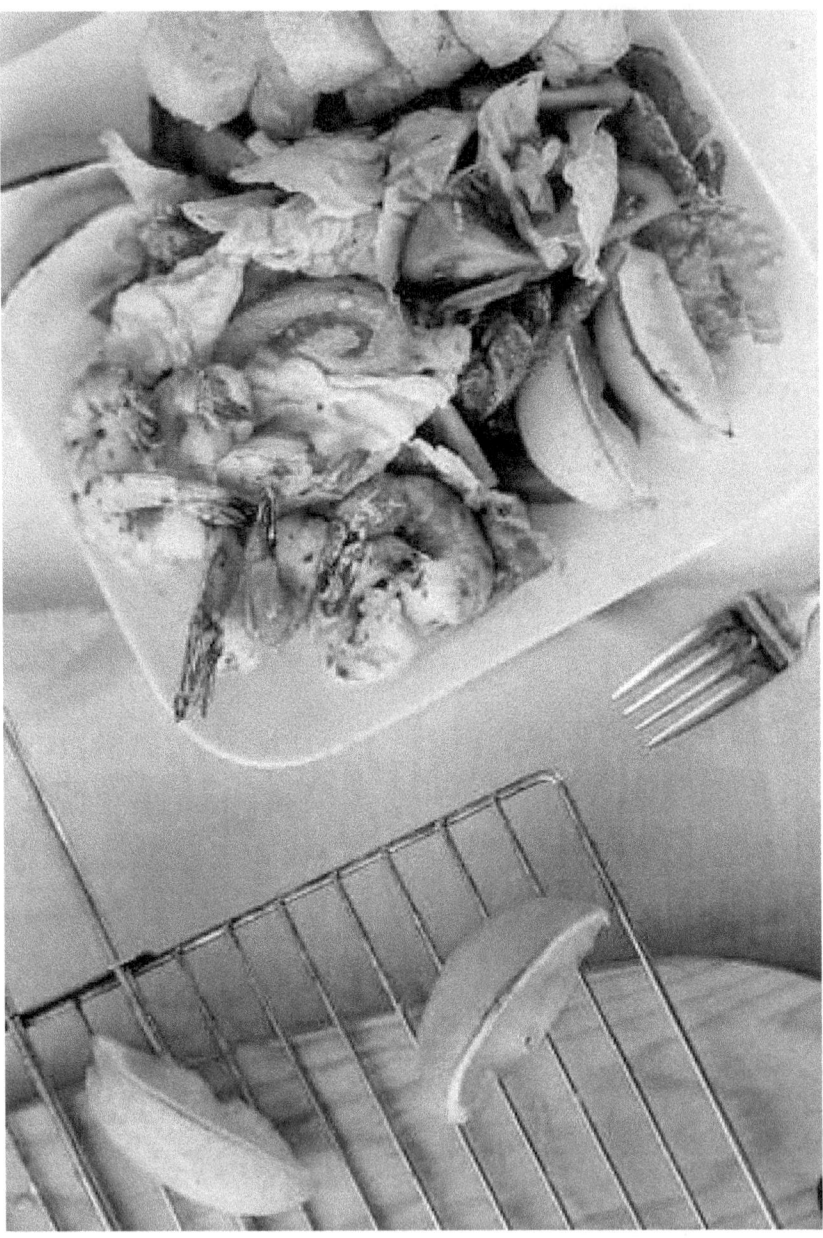

Table Of Content

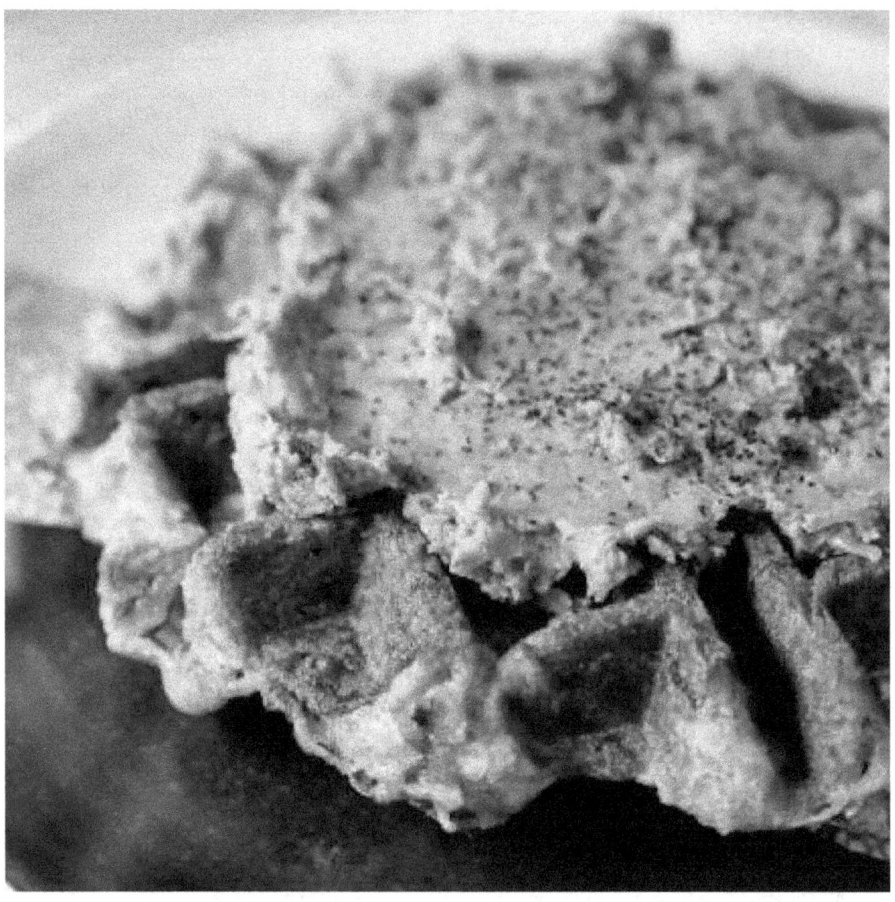

Additionally, the information in the following pages is intended only for informational purposes and should thus be thought of as universal. As befitting its nature, it is presented without assurance regarding its prolonged validity or interim quality. Trademarks that are mentioned are done without written consent and can in no way be considered an endorsement from the trademark holder.

CHAPTER 1: **BREAKFAST**

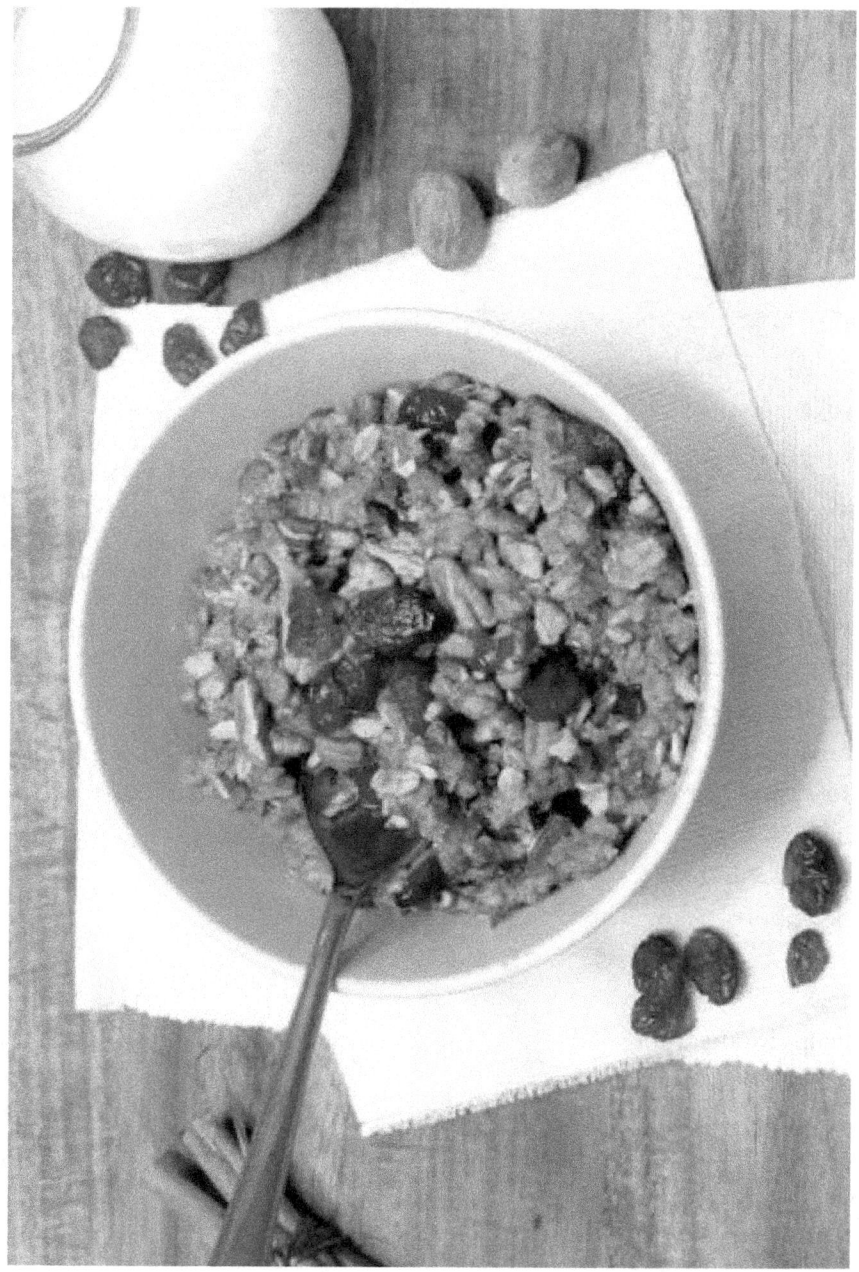

Baked Oatmeal

Prep:

10 mins

Cook:

40 mins

Total:

50 mins

Servings:

8

Yield:

8 servings

Ingredients

3 cups rolled oats

¾ cup brown sugar

2 teaspoons ground cinnamon (such as McCormick® Roasted Saigon Cinnamon)

1 teaspoon salt

1 cup milk

½ cup melted butter

2 teaspoons baking powder

2 eggs

2 teaspoons vanilla extract

¼ cup dried cranberries

¼ cup maple syrup

Directions

1

Preheat oven to 350 degrees F. Grease an 8x8-inch baking dish.

2

Mix oats, brown sugar, cinnamon, baking powder, and salt together in a bowl. Beat in milk, butter, maple syrup, eggs, and vanilla extract; fold in cranberries. Spread mixture into the prepared baking dish.

3

Bake in the preheated oven until bubbling, about 40 minutes.

Nutrition

Per Serving: 344 calories; protein 6.7g; carbohydrates 46g; fat 15.4g; cholesterol 79.4mg; sodium 531mg.

Sunrise Smoothies

Prep:

15 mins

Total:

15 mins

Servings:

2

Yield:

2 servings

Ingredients

½ cup orange juice

1 teaspoon white sugar

1 banana, frozen and chunked

½ cup honeydew melon, cubed

1 (8 ounce) container orange yogurt

1 peach, peeled and sliced

½ cup ice

Directions

1

Combine the orange juice, banana, peach, honeydew melon, yogurt, sugar, and ice in a blender. Blend until smooth, or chunky, as desired. Pour into two glasses and serve.

Nutrition

Per Serving: 239 calories; protein 5.8g; carbohydrates 52g; fat 1.3g; cholesterol 9mg; sodium 67.4mg.

Sweet Potato Cakes

Prep:

10 mins

Cook:

25 mins

Additional:

30 mins

Total:

1 hr 5 mins

Servings:

12

Yield:

12 servings

Ingredients

2 ¾ cups all-purpose flour

1 cup white sugar

¼ cup sweet potato puree

2 teaspoons ground cinnamon

½ teaspoon salt

¼ teaspoon ground cloves

1 ¾ cups cooled coffee

1 ½ teaspoons baking powder

¾ cup olive oil

Icing:

1 cup confectioners' sugar

1 teaspoon vanilla extract

¼ teaspoon ground cinnamon

1 tablespoon orange juice

Directions

1

Preheat the oven to 350 degrees F. Grease a 9x13-inch baking pan.

2

Combine flour, sugar, cinnamon, baking powder, salt, and cloves in a bowl and mix well. Add cooled coffee, oil, and sweet potato puree; mix well. Pour batter evenly into the prepared baking pan.

3

Bake in the preheated oven until a toothpick inserted in the center comes out clean, 25 to 30 minutes. Remove and allow to cool on a wire rack, about 30 minutes.

4

Stir together 1 cup confectioners' sugar, 1 tablespoon orange juice, vanilla extract, and cinnamon in a bowl. Add more sugar or orange juice, if needed, to achieve your desired consistency. Drizzle icing over the top of the cooled cake.

Nutrition

Per Serving: 336 calories; protein 3.1g; carbohydrates 50.4g; fat 13.8g; sodium 163.7mg.

Quinoa Pancakes

Prep:

10 mins

Cook:

5 mins

Total:

15 mins

Servings:

10

Yield:

10 servings

Ingredients

1 ½ cups quinoa flour

2 tablespoons honey

1 ½ teaspoons baking powder

½ teaspoon salt

3 eggs, beaten

2 tablespoons butter, melted

1 ¼ cups flaxseed milk

Directions

1

Grease a griddle or large skillet and preheat over medium heat.

2

Stir quinoa flour, baking powder, and salt together in a bowl. Stir flaxseed milk, eggs, melted butter, and honey into the flour mixture until you have a thin batter.

3

Pour 1/4 cup batter onto your hot cooking surface per pancake and cook until bubbles form on top, 2 to 3 minutes. Flip the pancake and cook until browned on the bottom, about 2 minutes more.

Nutrition

Per Serving: 138 calories; protein 4.9g; carbohydrates 17.3g; fat 5.6g; cholesterol 61.9mg; sodium 241.1mg.

Honey-Ginger Kale Salad

Prep:

30 mins

Total:

30 mins

Servings:

6

Yield:

6 servings

Ingredients

2 tablespoons cider vinegar

2 (10 ounce) bunches lacinato kale, stems removed, leaves thinly sliced

1 ½ teaspoons low-sodium soy sauce

1 ½ teaspoons grated fresh ginger

2 tablespoons olive oil

1 ½ tablespoons fresh orange juice

1 ½ teaspoons honey

Directions

1

Whisk together vinegar, juice, soy sauce, honey, and ginger in a small bowl. Add oil slowly, whisking constantly until incorporated.

2

Put kale in a large bowl. Drizzle with dressing, and mix well. Using your hands, massage kale until softened, wilted, and reduced in volume by about half.

Nutrition

Per Serving: 89 calories; protein 2.8g; carbohydrates 10g; fat 5.1g; sodium 110.9mg.

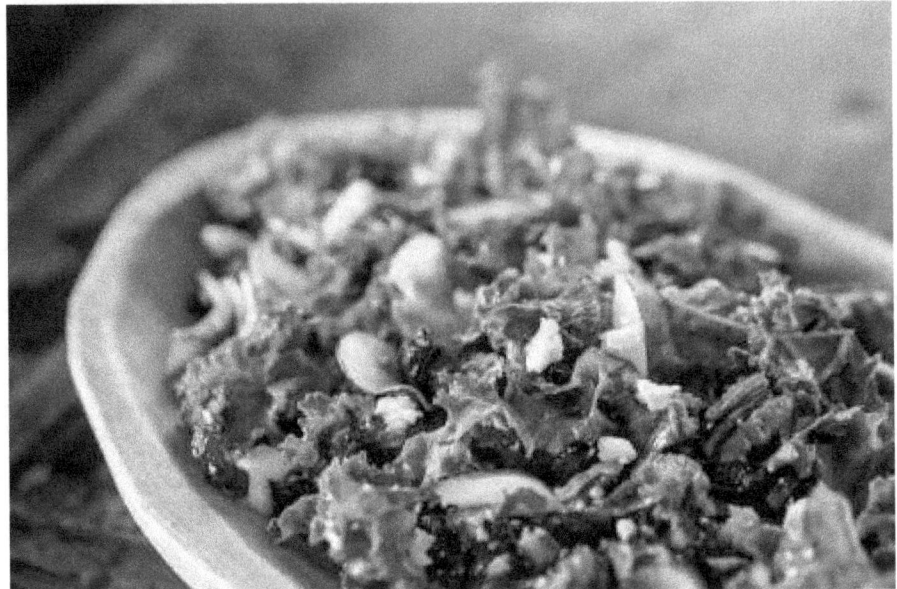

Greek Pita Pockets

Prep:

15 mins

Cook:

10 mins

Total:

25 mins

Servings:

4

Yield:

4 servings

Ingredients

½ cup Greek-style (thick) unflavored yogurt

⅔ cup Nikos® feta cheese crumbles

1 lemon, juiced

4 ounces bulk pork sausage

1 small onion, diced

¾ cup wild mushrooms, chopped

1 cup fresh baby spinach leaves, packed

⅓ cup Greek olives, diced

6 eggs, beaten

2 pitas, halved crosswise

Directions

1

In small bowl, stir together yogurt and lemon juice; set aside.

2

In nonstick skillet over medium-high heat, cook sausage, stirring frequently and crumbling for 2 minutes. Add onion, olives, and mushrooms; cook 4 minutes more.

3

Add spinach leaves and cook until wilted and sausage is fully cooked, about 1 to 3 minutes. Add eggs and cook, stirring constantly until almost dry. Remove from heat and stir in feta.

4

Stuff each pita half with feta-egg mixture. Serve immediately with lemon yogurt.

Nutrition

Per Serving: 382 calories; protein 21g; carbohydrates 23.4g; fat 23.4g; cholesterol 317.3mg; sodium 895.8mg.

Blackberry Banana Protein Shake

Prep:

5 mins

Total:

5 mins

Servings:

1

Yield:

1 protein shake

Ingredients

2 cups almond milk

¾ cup fresh blackberries

1 banana

1 cup vanilla Greek yogurt

Directions

1

Combine almond milk, yogurt, ice cubes, blackberries, and banana in a blender; blend until smooth.

Nutrition

Per Serving: 417 calories; protein 17.4g; carbohydrates 60g; fat 13.1g; cholesterol 18.7mg; sodium 379.4mg.

Protein Bowl

Prep:

5 mins

Total:

5 mins

Servings:

1

Yield:

1 serving

Ingredients

¼ cup Greek yogurt
½ chocolate protein bar, cut into small pieces
5 fresh strawberries, sliced
1 tablespoon peanut butter

Directions

1

Combine Greek yogurt and peanut butter in a bowl and whip together until smooth. Top with protein bar pieces and strawberries.

Nutrition

Per Serving: 305 calories; protein 12.9g; carbohydrates 34.6g; fat 14g; cholesterol 11.3mg; sodium 140.5mg.

Zucchini Waffles

15 mins

Cook:

5 mins

Total:

20 mins

Servings:

8

Yield:

8 waffles

Ingredients

2 eggs
1 tablespoon vegetable oil
1 pinch salt
½ cup dry potato flakes
¼ teaspoon onion powder
¼ teaspoon baking powder
3 cups shredded zucchini

Directions

1

Preheat a waffle iron according to manufacturer's instructions.

2

Mix zucchini, eggs, vegetable oil, onion powder, and salt together in a bowl. Stir in potato flakes and baking powder; mix until batter is combined.

3

Pour 1/2 cup of the batter onto the center of the waffle iron. Close the lid; cook until iron stops steaming and waffle is crisp, about 5 minutes.

Nutrition

Per Serving: 51 calories; protein 2.4g; carbohydrates 4.2g; fat 3g; cholesterol 46.5mg; sodium 59.9mg.

Quinoa Crepes

Prep:

15 mins

Cook:

10 mins

Total:

25 mins

Servings:

3

Yield:

3 servings

Ingredients

1 cup quinoa flour
2 large eggs
1 cup almond milk
1 teaspoon honey
2 tablespoons melted butter
1 pinch sea salt

Directions

1

Whisk quinoa flour, almond milk, eggs, honey, and sea salt together in a bowl until batter is smooth. Stir butter into batter.

2

Heat a lightly greased a skillet or griddle over medium-low heat. Pour 1/4 cup batter into the skillet and immediately rotate the skillet until the batter evenly coats the bottom in a thin layer. Cook until the top of the crepe is no longer wet and the bottom has turned light brown, about 2 minutes. Run a spatula around the edge of the skillet to loosen; flip crepe and cook until the other side has turned light brown, about 30 seconds. Repeat with remaining batter.

Nutrition

Per Serving: 312 calories; protein 11.2g; carbohydrates 32.2g; fat 15.1g; cholesterol 144.4mg; sodium 270.6mg.

Mediterranean Frittata

Prep:

15 mins

Cook:

40 mins

Additional:

10 mins

Total:

1 hr 5 mins

Servings:

4

Yield:

4 servings

Ingredients

3 sun-dried tomato halves

5 cloves garlic, minced

½ cup frozen chopped spinach

2 tablespoons shredded Parmesan cheese

1 (4.5 ounce) can sliced mushrooms with pieces, drained

3 ounces crumbled reduced-fat feta cheese

2 teaspoons extra-virgin olive oil

¼ yellow onion, minced

6 egg whites

¼ teaspoon salt

¼ teaspoon ground black pepper

¼ teaspoon dried basil

¼ cup skim milk

Directions

1

Preheat oven to 350 degrees F. Grease an 8-inch round pan.

2

Place sun-dried tomatoes into a bowl of warm water until rehydrated, about 10 minutes. Drain and chop.

3

Heat olive oil in a small skillet over medium heat; cook and stir onion and garlic until onion is translucent, about 10 minutes. Add spinach; cook and stir until thawed and water is evaporated, about 5 minutes. Stir in mushrooms, sun-dried tomatoes, and feta cheese until well mixed.

4

Whisk egg whites, skim milk, salt, pepper, and basil together in a bowl until very frothy. Carefully stir spinach mixture and 1 tablespoon Parmesan cheese into egg mixture. Pour into the prepared pan; top with remaining Parmesan cheese.

5

Bake in the preheated oven until frittata is set and browned on top, about 25 minutes.

Nutrition

Per Serving: 176 calories; protein 16.1g; carbohydrates 18.3g; fat 6.2g; cholesterol 10mg; sodium 1145.8mg.

Western Omelet

Prep:

15 mins

Cook:

5 mins

Total:

20 mins

Servings:

1

Yield:

1 omelet

Ingredients

2 teaspoons butter, divided
¼ cup chopped green bell pepper
2 green onions, sliced on the bias
salt and ground black pepper to taste
2 eggs
¼ cup cooked ham strips

Directions

1

Melt 1 teaspoon butter in a small skillet over medium heat. Add mushrooms, bell pepper, and green onions; cook until tender, about 5 minutes. Stir in ham until heated through, about 1 minute. Season with salt and pepper. Set filling mixture aside in a small bowl and keep warm.

2

Beat eggs together in a bowl; season with salt and pepper.

3

Heat the same skillet over medium-high heat. Add remaining 1 teaspoon butter; heat until foaming. Pour in eggs and cook for 30 seconds. Lift the edges of the omelet so that the uncooked egg runs under the cooked edges and comes into contact with the hot skillet. Shake and tilt the skillet to move the uncooked egg. Repeat until the top is set but still moist and soft, about 2 minutes.

4

Spread the filling over one side of the omelet. Fold the other half over the filling and slide omelet onto a plate.

Nutrition

Per Serving: 320 calories; protein 20.5g; carbohydrates 5.5g; fat 24.5g; cholesterol 412.4mg; sodium 793.1mg.

Banana & Cinnamon Cake

Prep:

15 mins

Cook:

35 mins

Additional:

1 hr

Total:

1 hr 50 mins

Servings:

12

Yield:

12 servings

Ingredients

Cake:

1 (18.25 ounce) package vanilla cake mix

1 cup water

3 eggs

⅓ cup oil

3 very ripe bananas, mashed

2 teaspoons ground cinnamon

1 teaspoon baking soda

Frosting:

1 cup milk

1 (3.5 ounce) package instant banana cream pudding mix

1 (8 ounce) container low-fat frozen whipped topping (such as Cool Whip® Lite), thawed

Directions

1

Preheat oven to 350 degrees F (175 degrees C). Grease a 13x9-inch baking dish.

2

Beat cake mix, water, eggs, and oil together in a bowl using a electric mixer until batter is smooth and well mixed, about 2 minutes. Mix bananas, cinnamon, and baking soda together in a separate bowl; stir into batter. Pour batter into the prepared baking dish.

3

Bake in the preheated oven until a toothpick inserted in the center of the cake comes out clean, 35 to 40 minutes. Cool cake completely.

4

Beat milk and pudding mix together in a bowl until smooth; fold in whipped topping until frosting is smooth. Spread frosting onto cooled cake.

Nutritions

Per Serving: 351 calories; protein 4.6g; carbohydrates 56g; fat 13.4g; cholesterol 48.1mg; sodium 534.8mg.

Pineapple Oatmeal

Prep:

15 mins

Cook:

25 mins

Additional:

5 mins

Total:

45 mins

Servings:

6

Yield:

6 servings

Ingredients

cooking spray

2 cups old-fashioned oats

½ teaspoon baking powder

½ teaspoon salt

¼ teaspoon baking soda

2 large eggs, lightly beaten

½ cup light coconut milk

⅓ cup melted butter

⅓ cup low-fat vanilla Greek yogurt

¼ cup honey

½ teaspoon vanilla extract

1 (8 ounce) can crushed pineapple, drained

½ cup shredded coconut

Directions

1

Preheat the oven to 350 degrees F (175 degrees C). Spray an 8-inch square dish with cooking spray and set aside.

2

Combine oats, baking powder, salt, and baking soda in a large bowl.

3

Whisk eggs, coconut milk, butter, yogurt, honey, and vanilla extract together in a separate bowl. Pour over the oats and stir until well combined. Fold in pineapple and coconut. Pour into the prepared baking dish.

4

Bake in the preheated oven until oatmeal has firmed up but not drying out, 25 to 30 minutes. Remove from the oven. Let cool for about 5 minutes before serving.

Nutritions

Per Serving: 340 calories; protein 7.4g; carbohydrates 41g; fat 17.2g; cholesterol 89.9mg; sodium 411.1mg.

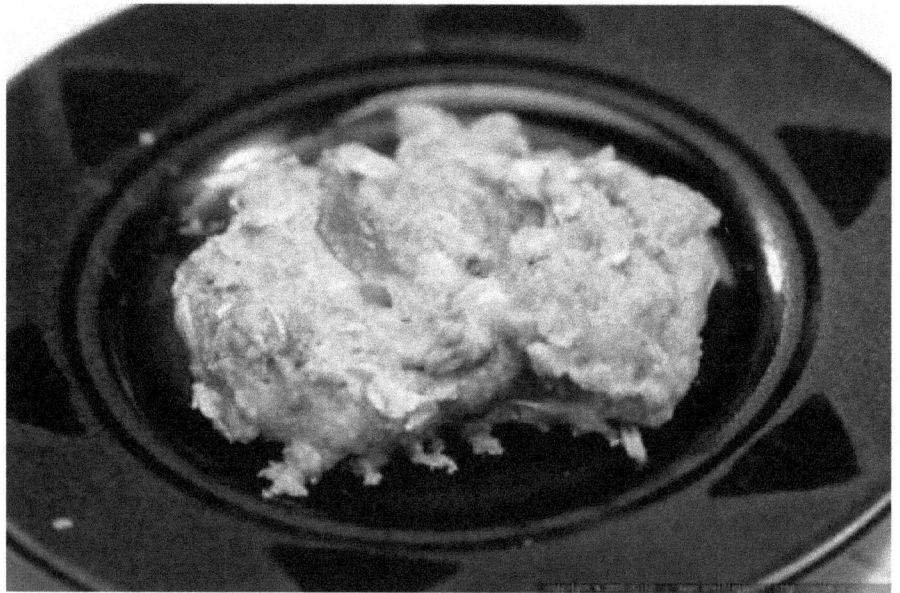

CHAPTER 2: LUNCH

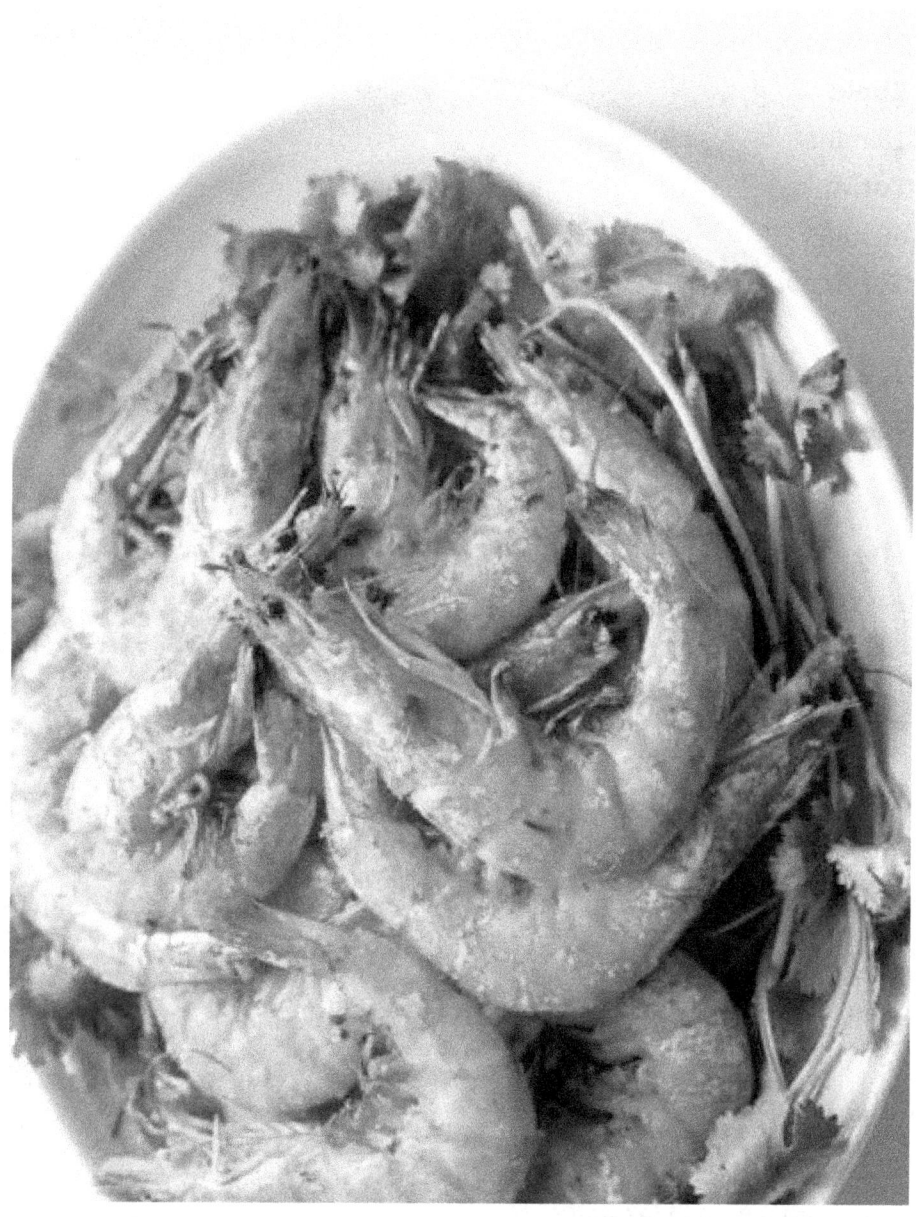

Salad with Shrimps

Prep:

30 mins

Cook:

10 mins

Total:

40 mins

Servings:

4

Yield:

4 servings

Ingredients

1 pound fresh asparagus, trimmed and sliced diagonally into 2-inch pieces

2 teaspoons white sugar

2 cups chopped tomatoes

½ cup diced green bell pepper

¼ cup finely chopped red onion

¼ cup tomato juice

3 tablespoons red wine vinegar

1 tablespoon olive oil

1 pound large peeled and deveined cooked shrimp

2 cups cubed and seeded English cucumber

2 cloves garlic, minced

⅛ teaspoon hot pepper sauce

1 pinch salt and ground black pepper to taste

8 cups mixed salad greens

¼ cup thinly sliced fresh basil

Directions

1

Place a steamer insert into a saucepan and fill with water to just below the bottom of the steamer. Bring water to a boil. Add asparagus, cover, and steam until crisp-tender, about 4 minutes. Drain and rinse in ice cold water; drain well.

2

Combine steamed asparagus, shrimp, cucumber, tomatoes, bell pepper, onion, and basil in a large bowl.

3

Combine tomato juice, vinegar, oil, garlic, sugar, hot sauce, salt, and pepper in a small bowl. Stir dressing with a whisk until well blended. Pour over shrimp mixture and toss well. Divide greens among 4 plates and top each with 2 cups of the shrimp salad.

Nutrition

Per Serving: 226 calories; protein 29.5g; carbohydrates 17.6g; fat 5.3g; cholesterol 221.3mg; sodium 374.1mg.

Scalloped Scallops

Prep:

10 mins

Cook:

20 mins

Total:

30 mins

Servings:

4

Yield:

4 servings

Ingredients

5 tablespoons butter, divided
salt and ground black pepper to taste
1 pound sea scallops
1 cup half-and-half
¾ cup milk
½ cup bread crumbs
3 tablespoons all-purpose flour

Directions

1

Preheat oven to 400 degrees F. Butter an 8-inch square baking dish.

2

Melt 3 tablespoons butter in a saucepan over medium heat. Cook and stir scallops in melted butter until lightly browned, about 5 minutes. Stir flour into scallop mixture until dissolved, 2 to 3 minutes.

3

Gradually pour half-and-half and milk into scallop mixture, while stirring constantly until milk mixture is thickened, 6 to 10 minutes; season with salt and pepper. Pour scallop mixture into the prepared baking dish.

4

Place remaining 2 tablespoons butter in microwave-safe bowl and heat in microwave until melted, 10-20 seconds. Stir bread crumbs into melted butter until coated; sprinkle over scallop mixture.

5

Bake in the preheated oven until bread crumbs are browned, about 10 minutes.

Nutrition

Per Serving: 451 calories; protein 34.3g; carbohydrates 24.2g; fat 24.1g; cholesterol 132.7mg; sodium 610.1mg.

Lentil Soup

Prep:

20 mins

Cook:

6 hrs

Total:

6 hrs 20 mins

Servings:

10

Yield:

10 servings

Ingredients

7 cups water

1 pound cooked, smoked lean ham, cut into chunks

½ teaspoon dried thyme

1 (14.5 ounce) can low-sodium diced tomatoes, undrained

6 ounces sliced carrots

1 ¾ cups dried lentils, rinsed

8 ounces chopped onion

6 ounces chopped celery

5 cloves garlic, minced

½ teaspoon ground black pepper

1 bay leaf

Directions

1

Combine water, ham, tomatoes, lentils, onion, carrots, celery, garlic, pepper, salt, thyme, and bay leaf in a slow cooker.

2

Cover and cook on low until lentils and vegetables are as soft as you like, 6 to 8 hours. Remove bay leaf before serving.

Nutrition

Per Serving: 259 calories; protein 18g; carbohydrates 26.7g; fat 8.9g; cholesterol 25.4mg; sodium 736.5mg.

Green Beans with Shallots and Prosciutto

Prep:

5 mins

Cook:

10 mins

Total:

15 mins

Servings:

4

Yield:

4 servings

Ingredients

3 tablespoons unsalted butter, divided

2 ounces prosciutto, chopped

1 pound haricots verts (thin French green beans)

2 tablespoons water

2 shallots, thinly sliced

½ teaspoon salt

Directions

1

Melt 1 tablespoon butter in a large skillet over medium-high heat. Add shallots and prosciutto; cook until prosciutto begins to crisp, 3 to 4 minutes. Remove mixture to a plate and set aside.

2

Add remaining butter to the skillet and add haricots verts. Saute for 1 to 2 minutes, then add water and cover. Let green beans steam until most of the water is absorbed, about 5 minutes. Season with salt.

3

Remove green beans to a nice serving dish; top with the shallots and prosciutto.

Nutrition

Per Serving: 182 calories; protein 5.5g; carbohydrates 12.3g; fat 13.3g; cholesterol 35.4mg; sodium 576.2mg.

Avocado Salad

Servings:

2

Yield:

2 servings

Ingredients

2 medium avocados

1 pinch chili powder

2 small tomatoes, chopped

1 tablespoon chopped fresh cilantro, or to taste

½ tablespoon ground black pepper

1 (5 ounce) can light tuna (such as Century®)

salt to taste

Directions

1

Scoop out avocado contents and place in a bowl. Set aside shells.

2

Mix in tuna, tomatoes, cilantro, pepper, chili powder, and salt. Divide mixture between shells to serve.

Nutrition

Per Serving: 417 calories; protein 21.1g; carbohydrates 22g; fat 30.3g; cholesterol 18.9mg; sodium 133.6mg.

Red Pepper & Goat Cheese Frittata

Prep:

15 mins

Cook:

20 mins

Total:

35 mins

Servings:

4

Yield:

4 servings

Ingredients

2 tablespoons olive oil

1 cup diced roasted red peppers

2 tablespoons minced garlic

½ teaspoon minced fresh basil

⅓ cup heavy cream

salt and pepper to taste

6 small red potatoes, thinly sliced

½ cup crumbled goat cheese

6 eggs

Directions

1

Preheat the oven's broiler and set the oven rack about 6 inches from the heat source.

2

Heat the olive oil in a cast-iron skillet over medium heat, and spread the potatoes into the hot pan in an even layer. Cover the skillet, and cook the potatoes until they start to turn tender, about 10 minutes. Stir in the red peppers and garlic, and sprinkle with salt and pepper. Cook and stir the potato mixture until the garlic begins to soften, about 2 minutes, sprinkle on the basil, and cook the mixture, stirring occasionally, until the basil is cooked, about 2 more minutes.

3

Whisk the eggs and cream together in a bowl, and pour the egg mixture over the vegetables in the skillet. Sprinkle the top with goat cheese, cover the skillet, and reduce the heat to low. Cook until the eggs are set but not dry, 3 to 5 minutes. Uncover the skillet, and place it under the broiler until the top of the frittata has browned, about 2 minutes.

Nutrition

Per Serving: 501 calories; protein 19.4g; carbohydrates 46.3g; fat 27.5g; cholesterol 320mg; sodium 412.9mg.

Chicken Fajita

Prep:

5 mins

Cook:

15 mins

Additional:

30 mins

Total:

50 mins

Servings:

5

Yield:

10 fajitas

Ingredients

2 lime (2" dia)s limes, juiced
2 large yellow bell peppers
2 tablespoons olive oil
2 tablespoons fajita seasoning
2 large red bell peppers
10 (6 inch) flour tortillas, warmed
1 pound skinless, boneless chicken breast halves

Directions

1

Whisk lime juice, olive oil, and fajita seasoning together in a bowl and pour into a resealable plastic bag. Add chicken breasts, coat with the marinade, squeeze out excess air, and seal the bag. Marinate in the refrigerator for 30 minutes.

2

Preheat an outdoor grill for medium heat and lightly oil the grate.

3

Cut bell peppers in half and discard the inner membranes and seeds.

4

Remove chicken from the marinade and shake off excess. Discard the remaining marinade.

5

Place chicken and peppers (cut-sides down) on the preheated grill. Cook, turning occasionally, until chicken is no longer pink in the center and the juices run clear, and peppers have nice grill marks on them, about 15 minutes. An instant-read thermometer inserted into the center should read at least 165 degrees F.

6

Cut peppers and chicken into strips and serve on tortillas.

Nutrition

Per Serving: 402 calories; protein 25.7g; carbohydrates 46.1g; fat 12.9g; cholesterol 51.7mg; sodium 624.8mg.

Buckwheat Soup

Prep:

15 mins

Cook:

40 mins

Additional:

1 hr

Total:

1 hr 55 mins

Servings:

6

Yield:

6 servings

Ingredients

1 cup brown lentils

3 tablespoons extra-virgin olive oil

1 tablespoon olive oil

1 small onion, grated

2 bay leaves

4 ½ cups low-sodium vegetable broth, divided

¾ cup raw buckwheat groats

1 (9 ounce) package fresh baby spinach

1 small carrot, grated

Directions

1

Soak lentils in a bowl of cold water for 1 hour. Drain and set aside.

2

Heat oil in a Dutch oven or heavy-bottomed stew pot over medium heat. Add grated onion and carrot and saute until soft, 3 to 5 minutes. Add lentils and bay leaves and stir until coated with oil. Pour in 3 cups vegetable broth, stir, and bring to a boil. Leave at a slow boil for 10-12 minutes.

3

Reduce heat to a simmer and add buckwheat. Simmer until lentils are soft but not mushy and buckwheat is cooked through, about 25 minutes, adding remaining broth if needed. Remove from the heat and fold in fresh spinach until wilted. Remove bay leaves.

4

Serve hot with a 1/2 tablespoon olive oil drizzled on top of each portion.

Nutrition

Per Serving: 224 calories; protein 7.2g; carbohydrates 28.9g; fat 10g; sodium 191.7mg.

Glazed Chicken

Prep:

5 mins

Cook:

15 mins

Additional:

20 mins

Total:

40 mins

Servings:

4

Yield:

4 chicken breasts

Ingredients

⅓ cup balsamic vinegar

2 tablespoons white sugar

4 (4 ounce) skinless, boneless chicken breasts

½ cup chicken broth

1 clove garlic, crushed

1 teaspoon Italian seasoning

3 teaspoons olive oil

Directions

1

Whisk together the vinegar, chicken broth, sugar, garlic, and Italian seasoning in a small bowl. Put chicken in a shallow bowl and add marinade. Allow to marinate for 20 minutes, turning chicken halfway.

2

Heat oil in a large skillet over medium-high heat. Remove chicken from marinade and place in skillet, saving marinade. Cook chicken for 4 minutes on each side. Add remaining marinade and cook until chicken is no longer pink in the center and the juices run clear, and sauce has started to thicken and coat chicken, about 5 minutes more. An instant-read thermometer inserted into the center should read at least 165 degrees F.

Nutrition

Per Serving: 199 calories; protein 23.9g; carbohydrates 10g; fat 6.4g; cholesterol 65.4mg; sodium 207.1mg.

Vegetarian Chili

Prep:

15 mins

Cook:

1 hr

Total:

1 hr 15 mins

Servings:

8

Yield:

8 servings

Ingredients

1 tablespoon olive oil

1 tablespoon salt

½ medium onion, chopped

2 bay leaves

1 teaspoon ground cumin

3 (28 ounce) cans whole peeled tomatoes, crushed

2 tablespoons dried oregano

2 stalks celery, chopped

2 green bell peppers, chopped

2 jalapeno peppers, chopped

3 cloves garlic, chopped

¼ cup chili powder

1 tablespoon ground black pepper

1 (15 ounce) can kidney beans, drained

1 (15 ounce) can garbanzo beans, drained

1 (15 ounce) can black beans

1 (15 ounce) can whole kernel corn

2 (4 ounce) cans chopped green chile peppers, drained

2 (12 ounce) packages vegetarian burger crumbles

Directions

1

Heat the olive oil in a large pot over medium heat. Stir in the onion, and season with bay leaves, cumin, oregano, and salt. Cook and stir until onion is tender, then mix in the celery, green bell peppers, jalapeno peppers, garlic, and green chile peppers. When vegetables are heated through, mix in the vegetarian burger crumbles. Reduce heat to low, cover pot, and simmer 5 minutes.

2

Mix the tomatoes into the pot. Season chili with chili powder and pepper. Stir in the kidney beans, garbanzo beans, and black beans. Bring to a boil, reduce heat to low, and simmer 45 minutes. Stir in the corn, and continue cooking 5 minutes before serving.

Nutrition

Per Serving: 391 calories; protein 28.2g; carbohydrates 58.7g; fat 7.9g; sodium 2571.2mg.

Garden Salad

Prep:

20 mins

Total:

20 mins

Servings:

4

Yield:

4 servings

Ingredients

10 romaine lettuce leaves, chopped

1 tablespoon salt

4 tomatoes, chopped

1 large cucumber, sliced

1 onion, sliced

2 tablespoons lemon juice

1 tablespoon extra-virgin olive oil

½ cup fresh parsley, chopped

1 cup sour cream

Directions

1

Toss the romaine lettuce, tomatoes, cucumber, onion, and parsley together in a large bowl; season with salt. Drizzle the lemon juice and olive oil over the salad; stir. Add the sour cream and mix until evenly coated.

Nutrition

Per Serving: 206 calories; protein 4.2g; carbohydrates 14.3g; fat 15.9g; cholesterol 25.3mg; sodium 1789.5mg.

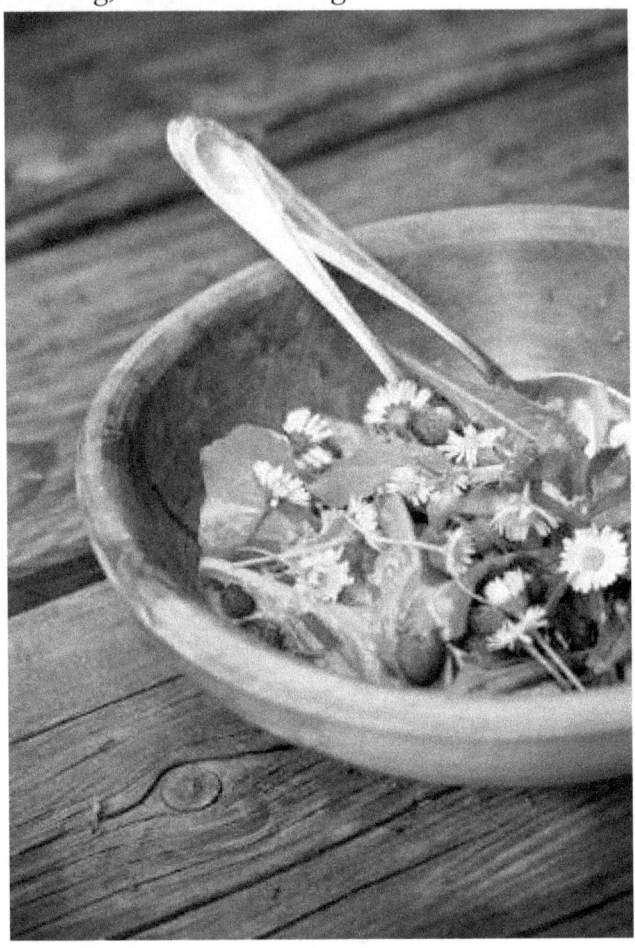

Chicken Scampi Pasta

Prep:

15 mins

Cook:

20 mins

Total:

35 mins

Servings:

3

Yield:

3 servings

Ingredients

1 (8 ounce) package spaghetti (such as Barilla® Spaghetti Rigati)

12 ounces jumbo shrimp, peeled and deveined

4 slices bacon, chopped

2 cloves garlic, minced

¼ cup chopped fresh parsley

⅛ teaspoon crushed red pepper flakes, or more to taste

½ cup chicken broth

½ cup heavy cream

⅓ cup freshly grated Parmesan cheese

salt and ground black pepper to taste

3 wedges fresh lemon

Directions

1

Bring a large pot of lightly salted water to a boil. Cook spaghetti in the boiling water, stirring occasionally, until nearly tender, about 8 minutes.

2

Meanwhile, cook bacon in a large skillet over medium heat until crisp, about 4 minutes. Drain on paper towels, leaving about 1 1/2 tablespoons grease in the skillet.

3

Add garlic to hot grease and cook until fragrant, about 30 seconds. Add shrimp and sprinkle with red pepper flakes. Cook until just cooked through and pink, about 2 minutes per side. Remove from the skillet and set aside.

4

Pour chicken broth into the hot skillet, and cook for about 1 minute. Stir in heavy cream, and bring to a simmer, about 2 minutes. Reduce heat to low, whisk in Parmesan cheese, and cook until sauce starts to thicken, about 2 minutes.

5

Drain spaghetti, reserving 1/2 cup of pasta water.

6

Return shrimp and bacon to the skillet and simmer until heated through, about 1 minute. Add spaghetti and toss all **Ingredients** together. Whisk in some of the reserved pasta water if sauce is too thick. Season with salt and pepper.

7

Garnish with chopped parsley and serve with a fresh lemon wedge to be squeezed over the pasta.

Nutrition

Per Serving: 615 calories; protein 37.3g; carbohydrates 60.1g; fat 24.5g; cholesterol 246.7mg; sodium 877.5mg.

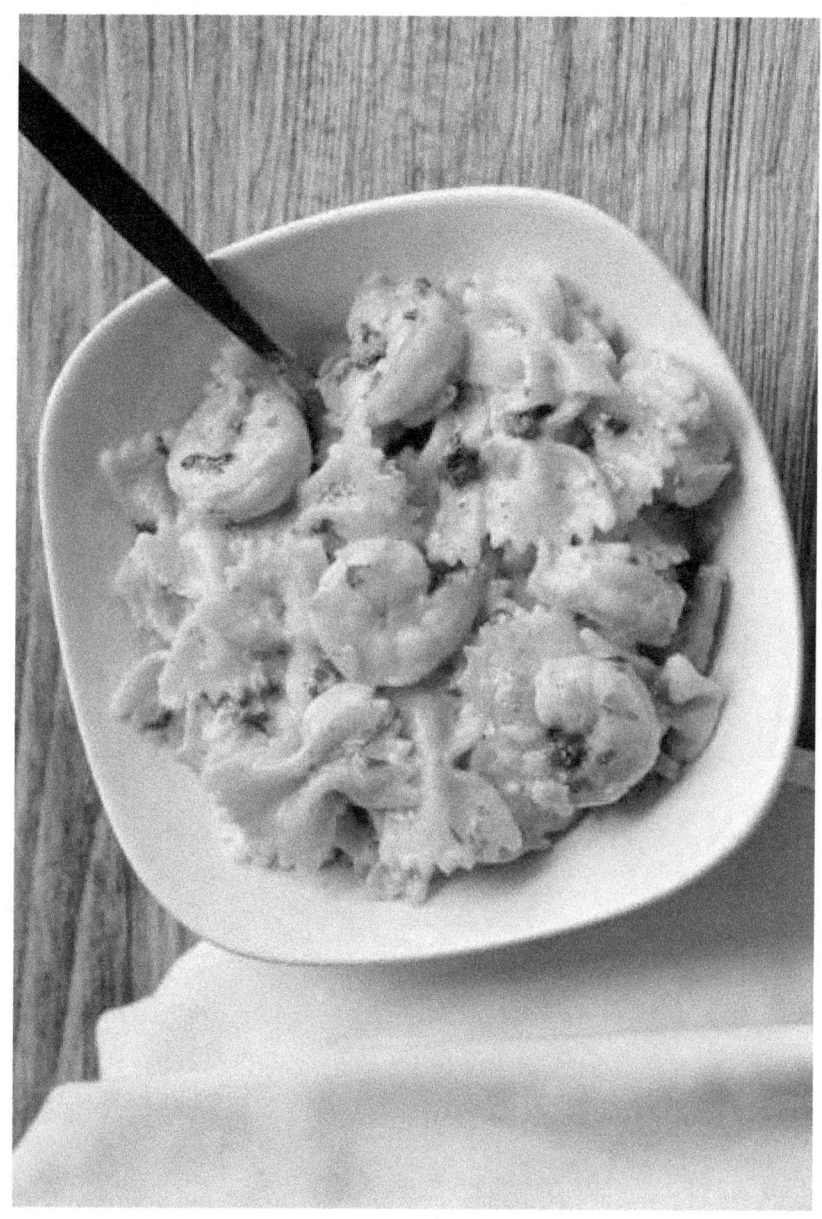

Lime Shrimp and Kale

Prep:

10 mins

Cook:

30 mins

Additional:

3 mins

Total:

43 mins

Servings:

2

Yield:

2 servings

Ingredients

1 bunch kale

2 tablespoons olive oil

1 tablespoon sriracha hot sauce

2 teaspoons lime juice

¼ teaspoon salt

Directions

1

Preheat oven to 300 degrees F (150 degrees C). Line 2 baking sheets with baking parchment.

2

Wash kale. Remove and discard ribs. Dry leaves thoroughly, using a salad spinner if available. Make sure no moisture remains. Tear kale leaves into 2- to 3-inch pieces.

3

Blend olive oil, Sriracha hot sauce, lime juice, and salt together with a whisk in a large bowl; add kale and toss to coat.

4

Divide kale onto prepared baking sheets and arrange so there is no overlapping of pieces.

5

Bake in preheated oven for 15 minutes, flip any pieces getting too browned on the bottom, and continue baking until the kale is crisp, about 15 minute more. Let kale chips cool 3 to 4 minutes before serving.

Nutritions
Per Serving: 236 calories; protein 7.4g; carbohydrates 23.6g; fat 15.1g; sodium 704.9mg.

CHAPTER 3: DINNER

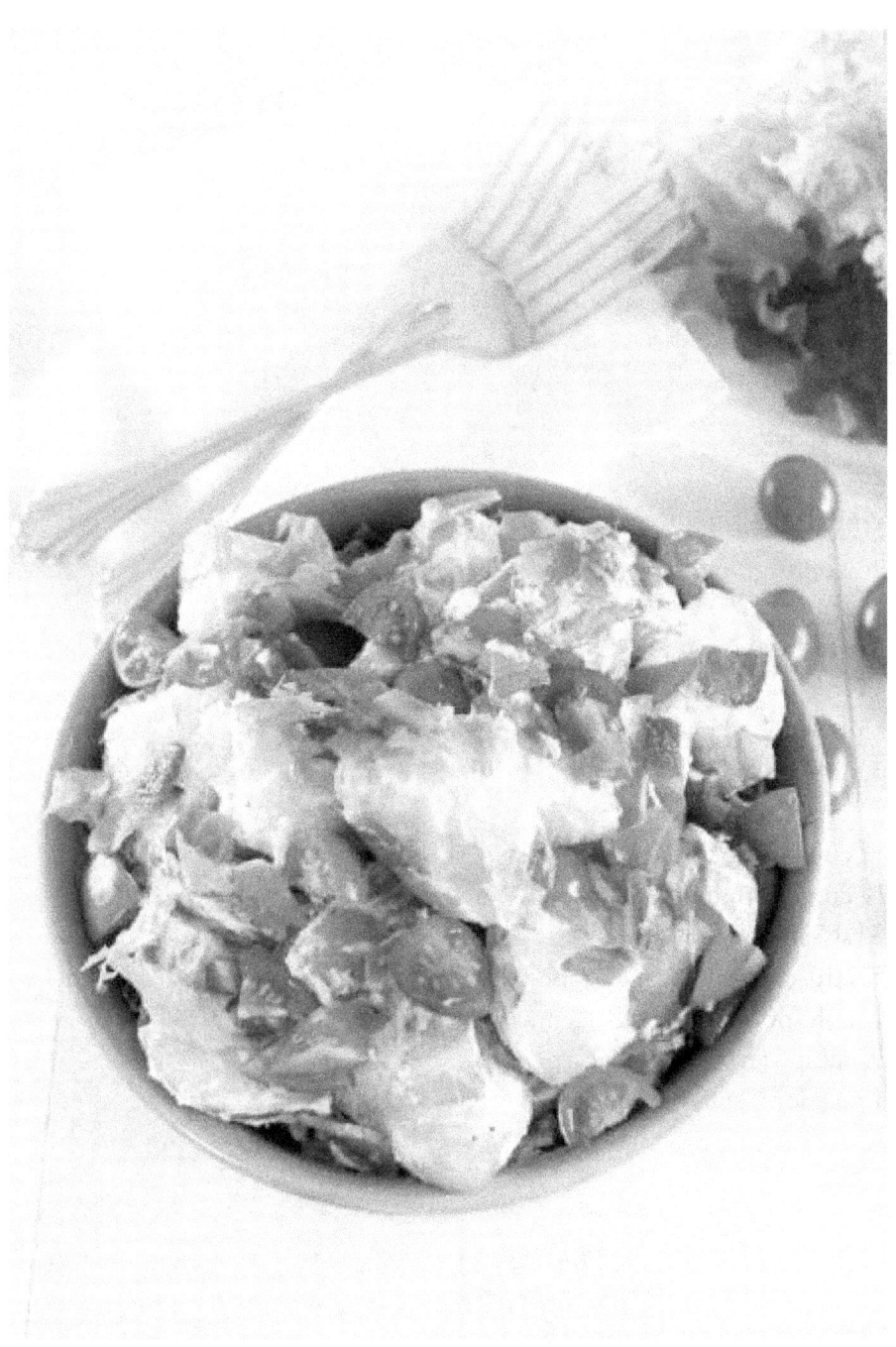

Potato Salad

Prep:

20 mins

Cook:

10 mins

Additional:

6 hrs

Total:

6 hrs 30 mins

Servings:

20

Yield:

20 servings

Ingredients

5 pounds red potatoes, chopped

3 cups mayonnaise

2 cups finely chopped pickles

½ cup chopped red onion

½ cup chopped celery

3 tablespoons prepared mustard

5 hard-cooked eggs, chopped

1 tablespoon apple cider vinegar

½ teaspoon ground black pepper

1 teaspoon salt, or to taste

Directions

1

Place potatoes into a large pot and cover with salted water; bring to a boil. Reduce heat to medium-low and simmer until tender, about 10 minutes. Drain. Return potatoes to empty pot to dry while you mix the dressing. Sprinkle with salt.

2

Stir mayonnaise, pickles, hard-cooked eggs, red onion, celery, mustard, cider vinegar, 1 teaspoon salt, and pepper together in a large bowl. Fold potatoes into the mayonnaise mixture. Allow to chill at least six hours, or overnight, before serving.

Nutrition

Per Serving: 339 calories; protein 4.1g; carbohydrates 20.4g; fat 27.6g; cholesterol 53.5mg; sodium 538.1mg.

Ginger Snapper

Prep:

10 mins

Cook:

20 mins

Total:

30 mins

Servings:

6

Yield:

6 servings

Ingredients

cooking spray

1 cup soy sauce

1 (2 inch) piece fresh ginger root, minced

¼ cup honey

2 cloves garlic, minced

1 (2 pound) whole snapper fillet

Directions

1

Preheat oven to 350 degrees F. Spray a large sheet of aluminum foil with cooking spray.

2

Thoroughly mix the soy sauce, honey, ginger, and garlic in a large bowl. Dip both sides of the fish into the soy sauce mixture, and place onto the aluminum foil. Spoon a little more sauce over the top of the fish. Roll up the aluminum foil to completely enclose the fillet.

3

Bake in the preheated oven until the fish is opaque and flakes easily, about 20 minutes.

Nutrition

Per Serving: 220 calories; protein 33.9g; carbohydrates 15.5g; fat 2.1g; cholesterol 55.5mg; sodium 2474.1mg.

Beef Brisket

Prep:

10 mins

Cook:

4 hrs

Total:

4 hrs 10 mins

Servings:

6

Yield:

6 servings

Ingredients

1 (3 pound) beef brisket, trimmed of fat
salt and pepper to taste
1 (12 fluid ounce) can beer
1 (12 ounce) bottle tomato-based chili sauce
1 medium onion, thinly sliced
¾ cup packed brown sugar

DirectionsInstructions Checklist

1

Preheat the oven to 325 degrees F.

2

Season the brisket on all sides with salt and pepper, and place in a glass baking dish. Cover with a layer of sliced onions. In a medium bowl, mix together the beer, chili sauce, and brown sugar. Pour over the roast. Cover the dish tightly with aluminum foil.

3

Bake for 3 hours in the preheated oven. Remove the aluminum foil, and bake for an additional 30 minutes. Let the brisket rest and cool slightly before slicing and returning to the dish. Reheat in the oven with the sauce spooned over the sliced meat.

Nutrition
Per Serving: 520 calories; protein 23.7g; carbohydrates 32.1g; fat 31g; cholesterol 92.1mg; sodium 142.2mg.

Pasta Primavera

Prep:

20 mins

Cook:

20 mins

Total:

40 mins

Servings:

4

Yield:

4 servings

Ingredients

2 cups whole grain penne pasta

½ cup freshly grated Parmesan cheese

1 tablespoon olive oil

½ cup chopped onion

2 cups sliced fresh mushrooms

1 small yellow summer squash, halved lengthwise and sliced

2 cups cherry tomatoes, halved

½ cup shredded carrot

1 pound fresh asparagus, trimmed and cut into 2-inch pieces

2 cloves garlic, minced

½ teaspoon ground black pepper

¼ teaspoon salt

⅛ teaspoon red pepper flakes

1 tablespoon chopped fresh oregano

Lemon wedges

Directions

1

Bring a large pot of lightly salted water to a boil. Add penne and cook, stirring occasionally, until tender yet firm to the bite, about 10 minutes.

2

Meanwhile, heat oil in an extra-large skillet over medium-high heat. Add onion; cook until softened, about 3 minutes. Add asparagus, mushrooms, and squash; cook until just tender, about 5 minutes. Add tomatoes, carrot, garlic, oregano, black pepper, salt, and red pepper flakes; cook until tomatoes begin to soften, about 1 minute.

3

Drain penne; stir into vegetable mixture along with 1/4 cup Parmesan cheese. Top servings with remaining cheese and serve with lemon wedges.

Nutrition
Per Serving: 281 calories; protein 15.8g; carbohydrates 41.5g; fat 7.7g; cholesterol 8.8mg; sodium 337.6mg

Grilled Cod

Prep:

10 mins

Cook:

10 mins

Additional:

15 mins

Total:

35 mins

Servings:

4

Yield:

4 servings

Ingredients

2 (8 ounce) fillets cod, cut in half

¼ teaspoon ground black pepper

1 tablespoon Cajun seasoning

½ teaspoon lemon pepper

¼ teaspoon salt

2 tablespoons chopped green onion (white part only)

2 tablespoons butter

1 lemon, juiced

Directions

1

Stack about 15 charcoal briquettes into a grill in a pyramid shape. If desired, drizzle coals lightly with lighter fluid and allow to soak for 1 minute before lighting coals with a match. Allow fire to spread to all coals, about 10 minutes, before spreading briquettes out into the grill; let coals burn until a thin layer of white ash covers the coals. Lightly oil the grates.

2

Season both sides of cod with Cajun seasoning, lemon pepper, salt, and black pepper. Set fish aside on a plate. Heat butter in a small saucepan over medium heat, stir in lemon juice and green onion, and cook until onion is softened, about 3-5 minutes.

3

Place cod onto oiled grates and grill until fish is browned and flakes easily, about 3 minutes per side; baste with butter mixture frequently while grilling. Allow cod to rest off the heat for about 5 minutes before serving.

Nutrition

Per Serving: 152 calories; protein 20.3g; carbohydrates 2.2g; fat 6.6g; cholesterol 63.4mg; sodium 660.6mg.

Taco Chicken Salad

Prep:

20 mins

Cook:

30 mins

Total:

50 mins

Servings:

4

Yield:

4 servings

Ingredients

1 ½ tablespoons paprika

1 ½ teaspoons cayenne pepper

1 ½ teaspoons garlic powder

1 teaspoon ground black pepper

1 teaspoon ground white pepper

¾ teaspoon ground cumin

1 ½ teaspoons onion powder

¾ teaspoon dried oregano

¾ teaspoon dried thyme

4 skinless, boneless chicken breast halves

1 tablespoon vegetable oil

4 tostada shells

¾ teaspoon salt

2 cups chopped romaine lettuce

2 cups fresh salsa

½ cup sliced black olives

½ cup ranch dressing

2 avocados - peeled, pitted, and sliced

½ cup shredded Cheddar cheese

Directions

1

Preheat oven to 350 degrees F.

2

Stir paprika, cayenne pepper, garlic powder, onion powder, black pepper, white pepper, cumin, oregano, thyme, and salt together in a bowl.

3

Rub spice mixture into each chicken breast to coat thoroughly.

4

Heat oil in a large skillet over high heat. Cook chicken breasts in hot oil until browned, about 5 minutes per side. Transfer chicken to a baking dish. Cover the dish with aluminum foil.

5

Bake in the preheated oven until chicken breasts are no longer pink in the center and the juices run clear, about 20 minutes. An instant-read thermometer inserted into the center should read at least 165 degrees F. Slice chicken into strips.

6

Fill each tostada shell with 1/2 cup lettuce. Divide chicken, salsa, avocados, Cheddar cheese, and olives between the tostada shells. Top each salad with ranch dressing.

Nutrition

Per Serving: 667 calories; protein 33.9g; carbohydrates 33.2g; fat 47g; cholesterol 87.6mg; sodium 1861.3mg.

Spicy Crackers

Prep:

20 mins

Cook:

35 mins

Additional:

15 mins

Total:

1 hr 10 mins

Servings:

18

Yield:

18 crackers

Ingredients

1 (12 ounce) package frozen riced cauliflower
cheese cloth
⅛ teaspoon cayenne pepper, or more to taste
1 cup shredded Parmesan cheese
1 egg
1 tablespoon dry ranch salad dressing mix

Directions

1

Place riced cauliflower in a microwave-safe bowl. Microwave, covered, for 3 to 4 minutes. Transfer to a cheesecloth-lined strainer and allow to cool for 15 minutes. Squeeze moisture out of the cooled riced cauliflower.

2

Preheat the oven to 425 degrees F. Line a baking sheet with parchment paper.

3

Combine riced cauliflower, egg, ranch mix, and cayenne pepper in a bowl and mix well. Stir in Parmesan cheese until incorporated.

4

Drop mixture with a small cookie scoop onto the prepared cookie sheet and flatten with a small hand rolling pin, a cup, or your hand to approximately 1/16-inch thickness. The thinner the dough, the crispier the cracker.

5

Bake crackers in the preheated oven for 10 minutes, flip, and bake for an additional 10 minutes. Cool on a wire rack.

Nutrition
Per Serving: 29 calories; protein 2.5g; carbohydrates 1.3g; fat 1.5g; cholesterol 14.2mg; sodium 103.5mg.

Lemon Swordfish

Prep:

15 mins

Cook:

20 mins

Total:

35 mins

Servings:

4

Yield:

4 servings

Ingredients

2 tablespoons skim milk

1 teaspoon dried basil leaves, crushed

3 tablespoons fresh lemon juice

1 teaspoon minced fresh parsley

1 teaspoon dried thyme, crushed

½ cup low-fat cottage cheese

4 (4 ounce) swordfish steaks

1 cup water

1 pound fresh steamed asparagus tips

1 bay leaf

Directions

1

In a blender or food processor, process the cottage cheese until creamy. Transfer the cottage cheese to a small bowl, and stir in the milk, 1 1/2 teaspoons of the lemon juice, parsley, basil, and 1/2 teaspoon of the dried thyme. Cover and chill in the refrigerator.

2

Preheat oven to 350 degrees F.

3

Place the fish in an 8x8 inch baking dish. Pour the water and the remaining lemon juice into the dish. Place the bay leaf in the water, and sprinkle the remaining 1/2 teaspoon of dried thyme over the fish. Cover the dish with foil.

4

Bake in a preheated oven for 20 minutes or until the fish flakes easily when tested with a fork and is opaque all the way through.

5

Meanwhile, place asparagus in a steamer over 1 inch of boiling water, and cover. Cook until tender but still firm, about 3 to 6 minutes. Drain.

6

When fish is done, transfer to a serving platter and arrange the asparagus next to the fish. Serve with the cottage cheese sauce.

Nutrition
Per Serving: 191 calories; protein 29g; carbohydrates 7.2g; fat 5.2g; cholesterol 46.1mg; sodium 221.6mg.

Citrus Swortfish

Prep:

10 mins

Cook:

15 mins

Additional:

30 mins

Total:

55 mins

Servings:

6

Yield:

6 servings

Ingredients

1 orange, peeled, sectioned, and cut into bite-size

1 ½ pounds swordfish steaks

½ cup canned pineapple chunks, undrained

2 jalapeno peppers, seeded and minced

3 tablespoons orange juice

1 tablespoon diced red bell pepper

2 teaspoons white sugar

¼ cup diced fresh mango

1 tablespoon chopped fresh cilantro

1 tablespoon olive oil

¼ teaspoon cayenne pepper

1 tablespoon pineapple juice concentrate, thawed

½ cup fresh orange juice

Directions

1

Make the salsa: In a medium-size bowl, combine oranges, pineapple chunks, mango, minced jalapenos, 3 tablespoons orange juice, diced red bell pepper, sugar, and cilantro. Mix well, and refrigerate covered.

2

In a non-reactive bowl, mix 1/2 cup orange juice, olive oil, cayenne pepper, and pineapple juice concentrate. Place swordfish steaks in bowl, and turn to coat well. Marinate the swordfish in the mixture for 30 minutes.

3

Prepare an outside grill with oiled rack set 6 inches from the heat source. On a gas grill, set the heat to medium-high.

4

Grill the swordfish on each side for a total time of about 13 to 15 minutes, until opaque in the center. Serve the grilled fish with the salsa.

Nutrition

Per Serving: 214 calories; protein 23.2g; carbohydrates 14g; fat 7g; cholesterol 44.3mg; sodium 103mg.

Coriander Pork

Prep:

5 mins

Total:

5 mins

Servings:

16

Yield:

1 cup

Ingredients

2 tablespoons kosher salt

2 tablespoons ground coriander

1 ½ teaspoons ground black pepper

4 tablespoons hot chili powder

1 tablespoon paprika

1 ½ teaspoons ground allspice

6 tablespoons ground cumin

Directions

1

Combine the kosher salt, coriander, cumin, chili powder, paprika, allspice, and black pepper in a bowl and mix thoroughly. Store in an airtight container at room temperature until ready to use.

2

To use, rub 1 tablespoon per serving onto the meat of your choice before grilling or cooking as desired.

Nutrition

Per Serving: 20 calories; protein 0.8g; carbohydrates 3g; fat 1.1g; sodium 744.4mg.

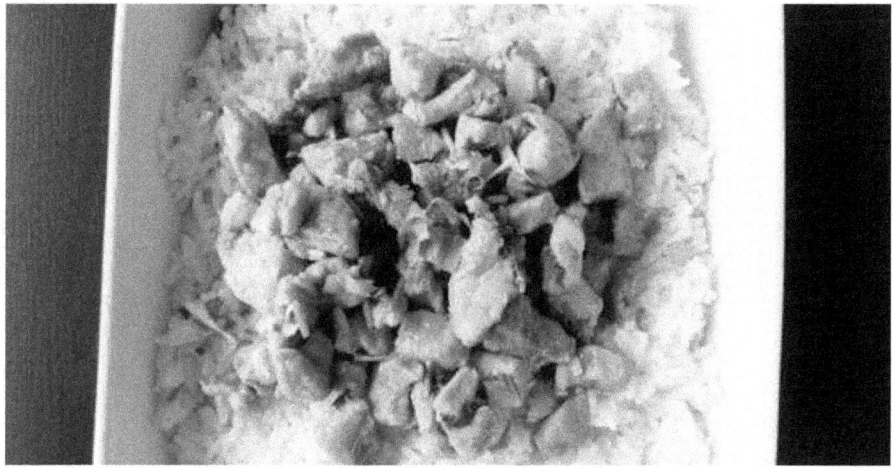

Caramelized Onions

Prep:

10 mins

Cook:

10 hrs

Total:

10 hrs 10 mins

Servings:

16

Yield:

1 quart

Ingredients

¼ cup melted butter, divided
1 teaspoon salt
8 onions, thinly sliced

Directions

1

Rub bottom and sides of slow cooker with 1/2 of the butter. Toss onions and salt with remaining butter in a bowl.

2

Cook onions on Low until browned and sweet, about 10 hours.

Nutrition

Per Serving: 71 calories; protein 1.3g; carbohydrates 10.6g; fat 3g; cholesterol 7.6mg; sodium 170.3mg.

Chickpea Meatballs

Prep:

20 mins

Cook:

30 mins

Total:

50 mins

Servings:

4

Yield:

4 servings

Ingredients

cooking spray
1 tablespoon salt-free seasoning blend
2 tablespoons olive oil
1 white onion, minced
6 cloves garlic, minced
¾ cup dry bread crumbs
1 egg
2 tablespoons parsley
2 cups canned chickpeas, drained
salt and ground black pepper to taste

Directions

1

Preheat oven to 375 degrees F. Grease a baking sheet with cooking spray.

2

Heat olive oil in a large skillet over medium heat. Add onion and garlic; cook and stir until tender, about 6 minutes.

3

Pulse chickpeas in a food processor until finely ground. Add onion and garlic, bread crumbs, egg, parsley, seasoning blend, salt, and black pepper; process until mixture holds together like a dough.

4

Scoop out 2 tablespoons of the mixture and roll into a ball; set on the prepared baking sheet. Repeat with remaining mixture.

5

Bake in the preheated oven until bottom is golden brown, about 15 minutes. Turn each meatball over and continue baking until golden brown on top, about 10 minutes more.

Nutrition

Per Serving: 331 calories; protein 11.2g; carbohydrates 48.7g; fat 10.6g; cholesterol 46.5mg; sodium 567.5mg.

Prunes Filling

Prep:

10 mins

Total:

10 mins

Servings:

24

Yield:

3 cups

Ingredients

1 cup chopped pecans
1 (16 ounce) can stewed prunes
2 tablespoons white sugar
½ teaspoon ground cinnamon
¼ teaspoon ground cloves
1 tablespoon lime juice

Directions

1

Chop pecans and prunes together in a blender or food processor, stir in the sugar, cinnamon, cloves and lime juice. Use as a filling for cookies or pastries.

Nutritions

Per Serving: 55 calories; protein 0.6g; carbohydrates 7g; fat 3.3g; sodium 0.6mg.

Bread Stick

Prep:

15 mins

Cook:

12 mins

Additional:

30 mins

Total:

57 mins

Servings:

12

Yield:

24 sticks

Ingredients

2 (8 ounce) packages refrigerated dinner roll dough

¼ cup margarine, melted

1 tablespoon garlic salt

¼ cup grated Parmesan cheese

2 tablespoons sesame seeds (Optional)

Directions

1

Lightly grease one large baking sheet.

2

Divide each roll in half. Roll dough between hands to make a 4-inch long stick. Place sticks on the prepared baking sheet. Brush lightly with egg white or melted butter or margarine. Sprinkle with garlic salt.

Sprinkle with parmesan cheese or sesame seeds. Cover and allow to rise until doubled in size, about 30 minutes.

3

Bake in a preheated 350 degrees F (175 degrees C) oven for 12 minutes or until golden brown. Do not overbake as these burn easily on the bottom.

Nutritions

Per Serving: 197 calories; protein 3.7g; carbohydrates 15.3g; fat 13g; cholesterol 1.5mg; sodium 815.8mg.

CHAPTER 4: SNACK & APPETIZER

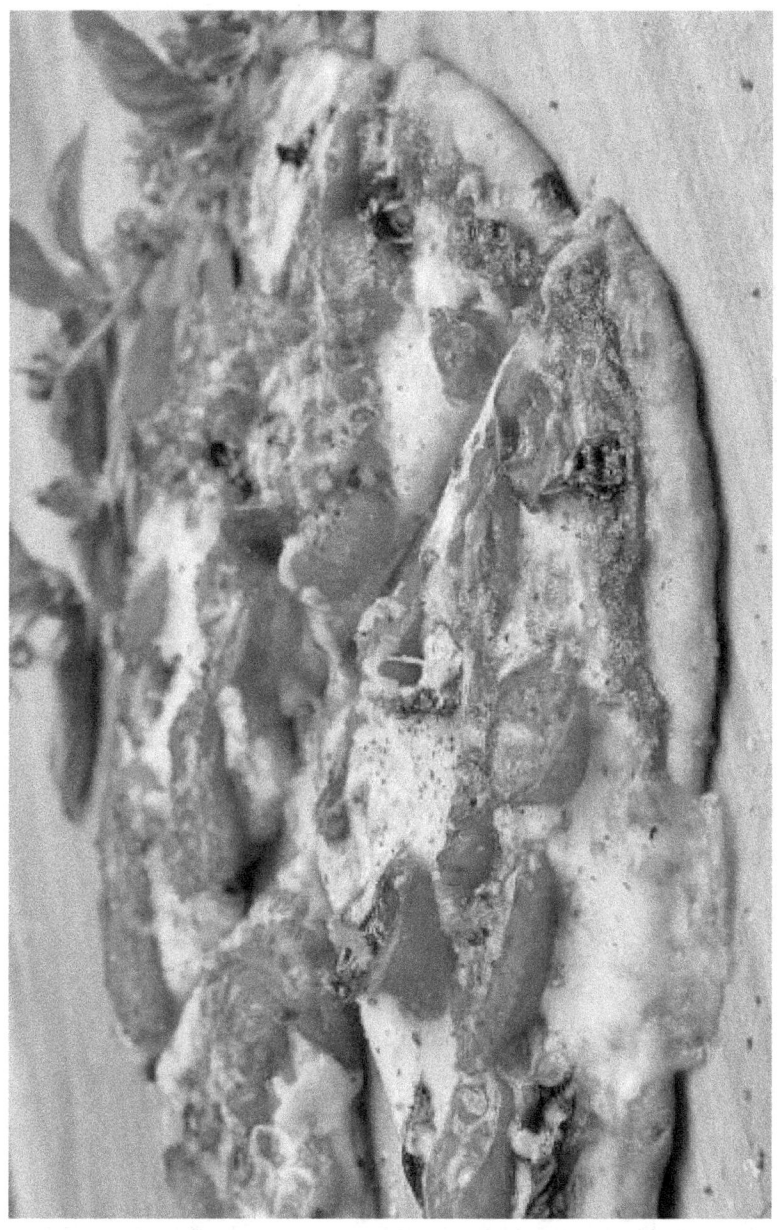

Pita Pizza

Prep:

5 mins

Cook:

15 mins

Total:

20 mins

Servings:

1

Yield:

1 serving

Ingredients

1 teaspoon olive oil

3 tablespoons pizza sauce

¼ cup sliced crimini mushrooms

⅛ teaspoon garlic salt

½ cup shredded mozzarella cheese

1 pita bread round

Directions

1

Preheat grill for medium-high heat.

2

Spread one side of the pita with olive oil and pizza sauce. Top with cheese and mushrooms, and season with garlic salt.

3

Lightly oil grill grate. Place pita pizza on grill, cover, and cook until cheese completely melts, about 5 minutes.

Nutrition

Per Serving: 405 calories; protein 19.7g; carbohydrates 39.9g; fat 18g; cholesterol 44.2mg; sodium 1155.9mg.

Pickled Asparagus

Prep:

10 mins

Cook:

5 mins

Total:

15 mins

Servings:

10

Yield:

1 quart

Ingredients

1 bunch fresh asparagus spears

2 tablespoons Old Bay Seasoning TM

2 bay leaves

1 cup water

1 cup white wine vinegar

¼ cup brown sugar

4 cloves garlic, crushed

6 whole black peppercorns

1 jalapeno pepper, seeded and julienned

4 sprigs fresh thyme

1 teaspoon salt

Directions

1

Trim the bottoms off of the asparagus, and pack loosely into a 1 quart jar.

2

Combine the water, white wine vinegar, brown sugar, garlic, jalapeno, thyme sprigs, bay leaves, salt and whole peppercorns in a saucepan. Bring to a boil, and boil hard for 1 minute.

3

Pour the hot liquid over the asparagus in the jar, filling to cover the tips of the asparagus. Cover, and cool to room temperature. Store in the refrigerator for 24 hours to blend flavors before serving.

Nutrition
Per Serving: 37 calories; protein 1.3g; carbohydrates 8.5g; fat 0.2g; sodium 564.9mg.

Almond Bars

Prep:

10 mins

Cook:

10 mins

Additional:

5 mins

Total:

25 mins

Servings:

48

Yield:

48 bars

Ingredients

12 graham crackers
1 teaspoon vanilla extract
¾ cup butter
1 cup brown sugar
1 cup sliced almonds

Directions

1

Preheat oven to 350 degrees F. Grease a 10x15 inch jelly roll pan.

2

Break graham crackers into 4 pieces and arrange them touching on the prepared jelly roll pan. Sprinkle the sliced almonds over the crackers.

In a small saucepan, melt butter. When butter is melted, stir in the brown sugar and vanilla until smooth and remove from heat. Pour the butter mixture evenly over the graham crackers in the pan.

3

Bake for 8 to 10 minutes in the preheated oven. Watch carefully so that the edges do not burn. Cut bars while still warm and remove from pan. If the bars are stuck, put the pan into the warm oven for a minute to loosen.

Nutrition

Per Serving: 63 calories; protein 0.7g; carbohydrates 6.1g; fat 4.2g; cholesterol 7.6mg; sodium 42.5mg.

Roasted Cashews

Prep:

15 mins

Cook:

10 mins

Total:

25 mins

Servings:

10

Yield:

10 servings

Ingredients

2 ½ cups unsalted cashews

2 tablespoons coarsely chopped fresh rosemary

1 tablespoon dark brown sugar

1 tablespoon kosher salt

1 teaspoon ground cayenne pepper

1 tablespoon margarine, melted

Directions

1

Preheat the oven to 375 degrees F.

2

Place cashews on a baking sheet.

3

Bake in the preheated oven until warmed through, about 10 minutes.

4

Stir rosemary, margarine, brown sugar, salt, and cayenne pepper together in a large bowl.

5

Pour warm cashews into the rosemary mixture and toss to coat. Serve warm or allow to cool and store in an airtight container.

Nutrition

Per Serving: 212 calories; protein 5.3g; carbohydrates 12.7g; fat 17g; sodium 808.1mg.

Surprize Watermelon

Prep:

20 mins

Additional:

1 hr

Total:

1 hr 20 mins

Servings:

12

Yield:

12 servings

Ingredients

6 cups cubed seeded watermelon

⅓ cup apple cider vinegar

½ red onion, cut into thin half-moon slices

½ teaspoon ground black pepper

2 tablespoons chopped fresh mint

Directions

1

Toss watermelon, red onion, apple cider vinegar, mint, and black pepper together in a large mixing bowl. Refrigerate until chilled completely, about 1 hour.

Nutrition

Per Serving: 26 calories; protein 0.5g; carbohydrates 6.3g; fat 0.1g; sodium 1.3mg.

Spaghetti Pie

Prep:

15 mins

Cook:

40 mins

Total:

55 mins

Servings:

12

Yield:

12 servings

Ingredients

1 (16 ounce) package spaghetti

2 cups cracker crumbs

1 cup grated Parmesan cheese

2 tablespoons chopped fresh parsley

1 tablespoon dried minced onion, divided

1 tablespoon garlic salt, divided

1 ½ sticks butter, melted

2 cups milk

4 eggs

Directions

1

Bring a large pot of lightly salted water to a boil. Cook spaghetti in the boiling water, stirring occasionally, until tender yet firm to the bite, about 12 minutes. Drain thoroughly.

2

Preheat the oven to 350 degrees F (175 degrees C). Thoroughly butter a 9x13-inch baking pan.

3

Layer 1/2 the cooked spaghetti into the bottom of the prepared pan. Sprinkle 1/2 the cracker crumbs, 1/2 the Parmesan cheese, 1/2 the parsley, 1/2 the minced onion, and 1/2 the garlic salt on top. Pour in 1/2 of the melted butter. Repeat with remaining spaghetti, cracker crumbs, Parmesan cheese, parsley, minced onion, garlic salt, and butter.

4

Mix milk and eggs together in a bowl. Pour over the spaghetti mixture.

5

Bake in the preheated oven until set, about 30 minutes. Cut pie in squares.

Nutritions

Per Serving: 389 calories; protein 12.9g; carbohydrates 46.1g; fat 16.8g; cholesterol 101.6mg; sodium 684.7mg.

Smoked Trout Spread

Prep:

10 mins

Cook:

5 hrs

Additional:

8 hrs 30 mins

Total:

13 hrs 40 mins

Servings:

6

Yield:

6 servings

Ingredients

2 pounds steelhead trout fillets
2 tablespoons olive oil
4 cloves garlic, chopped
1 ½ tablespoons dried rosemary, crushed
1 cup sugar-based curing mixture (such as Morton® Tender Quick®)
1 quart water
ground black pepper to taste
1 pound alder wood chips, soaked in water or wine

Directions

1

Rinse the fish fillets and place them in a shallow glass baking dish. Drizzle olive oil over the fish and season with garlic and rosemary. Rub the seasonings into the fish. Cover and refrigerate overnight.

2

Dissolve the curing salt in the water and pour into the dish with the fish. Let it marinate for 15 minutes per half inch of thickness.

3

Meanwhile, prepare your smoker for a four hour slow burn using charcoal. The temperature should be at 150 degrees F (65 degrees C) before you get started.

4

Remove the fish from the brine and discard leftover liquid. Place each piece of fish onto a small piece of aluminum foil - just big enough to hold the fillet, and season with pepper to taste. Place them on the rack in the smoker. Sprinkle a handful of the soaked wood chips over the coals or place in a heat box. Cover and allow fish to smoke for 2 hours, adding more wood chips as needed.

5

Increase the heat in the smoker (add more charcoal) to 200 degrees F (95 degrees C) and let the fish smoke until the internal temperature of the fillets reaches 165 degrees F (72 degrees C). Remove from the smoker and let rest for 20 minutes before serving.

Nutritions
Per Serving: 203 calories; protein 25.5g; carbohydrates 1.3g; fat 10.1g; cholesterol 125.6mg; sodium 18955.6mg.

CHAPTER 5: SMOOTHIES AND DRINKS

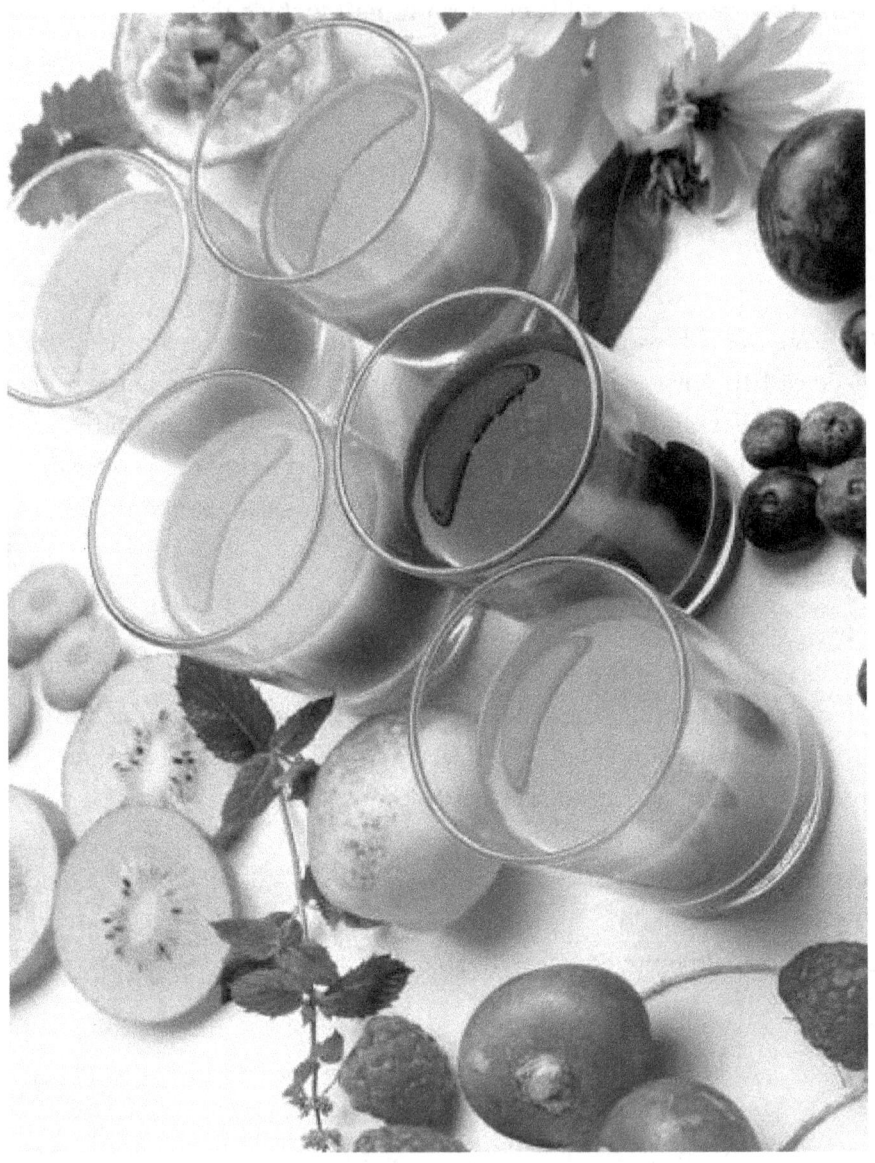

Healthy Coffee Smoothie

Prep:

5 mins

Total:

5 mins

Servings:

1

Yield:

1 smoothie

Ingredients

1 cup brewed coffee
2 tablespoons coconut oil, melted
2 large pasteurized egg yolks
1 tablespoon coconut sugar
¼ cup avocado
¼ cup ice cubes

Directions

1

Combine coffee, egg yolks, avocado, ice cubes, and coconut sugar in a blender; blend until smooth. Add coconut oil and blend until smooth.

Nutrition

Per Serving: 486 calories; protein 6.7g; carbohydrates 19.4g; fat 44.5g; cholesterol 409.7mg; sodium 30.4mg.

Banana and Almond Muffin

Prep:

10 mins

Cook:

20 mins

Total:

30 mins

Servings:

20

Yield:

20 muffins

Ingredients

6 large ripe bananas

2 teaspoons baking powder

1 cup brown sugar

¾ cup salted butter, melted

2 eggs

1 ½ cups all-purpose flour

1 ¼ cups whole wheat flour

½ cup ground flax seeds

½ cup white sugar

2 teaspoons baking soda

Directions

1

Preheat oven to 350 degrees F. Line 2 muffin tins with paper liners.

2

Mash bananas in a bowl. Add brown sugar, butter, white sugar, and eggs; mix well. Add all-purpose flour, whole wheat flour, flax seeds, baking soda, and baking powder. Scoop batter into the prepared tins.

3

Bake in the preheated oven until tops spring back when lightly pressed, about 20 minutes.

Nutrition

Per Serving: 240 calories; protein 3.7g; carbohydrates 38.7g; fat 8.9g; cholesterol 36.9mg; sodium 235.5mg.

Pumpkin Smoothie

Prep:

10 mins

Total:

10 mins

Servings:

2

Yield:

2 glasses

Ingredients

½ cup pumpkin puree
6 ice cubes
1 scoop vanilla protein powder
1 cup light vanilla soy milk
½ teaspoon ground cinnamon
1 small banana

Directions

1

Combine vanilla soy milk, pumpkin puree, ice, banana, vanilla protein powder, and ground cinnamon in a blender; blend until smooth.

Nutrition

Per Serving: 191 calories; protein 22.9g; carbohydrates 23.1g; fat 1.9g; cholesterol 6.3mg; sodium 314.6mg.

Kiwi Juice

Prep:

10 mins

Cook:

30 mins

Additional:

12 hrs

Total:

12 hrs 40 mins

Servings:

40

Yield:

5 cups

Ingredients

24 kiwis, peeled and mashed

4 cups white sugar

¼ cup fresh lemon juice

3 apples, unpeeled and halved

¾ cup pineapple juice

Directions

1

In a large saucepan, combine 3 cups mashed kiwi, pineapple juice, lemon juice and apples. Bring to a boil and then add the sugar; stir to dissolve, reduce heat and simmer for 30 minutes.

2

Sterilize the jars and lids in boiling water for at least 5 minutes. Pack the jam into the hot, sterilized jars, filling the jars to within 1/4 inch of the top. Run a knife or a thin spatula around the insides of the jars after they have been filled to remove any air bubbles. Wipe the rims of the jars with a moist paper towel to remove any food residue. Top with lids, and screw on rings.

3

Place a rack in the bottom of a large stockpot and fill halfway with water. Bring to a boil over high heat, then carefully lower the jars into the pot using a holder. Leave a 2 inch space between the jars. Pour in more boiling water if necessary until the water level is at least 1 inch above the tops of the jars. Bring the water to a full boil, cover the pot, and process for 10 minutes.

Nutrition

Per Serving: 113 calories; protein 0.6g; carbohydrates 28.7g; fat 0.3g; sodium 1.5mg.

Strawberry and Banana Shake

Prep:

5 mins

Total:

5 mins

Servings:

2

Yield:

2 cups

Ingredients

1 cup skim milk

1 scoop vanilla-flavored whey protein powder

2 cups ice

1 cup strawberries

1 large banana

1 tablespoon natural peanut butter

Directions

1

Layer milk, protein powder, ice, strawberries, banana, and peanut butter in a blender in this order; blend until creamy and smooth.

Nutritions

Per Serving: 261 calories; protein 26.1g; carbohydrates 31.1g; fat 5.2g; cholesterol 8.7mg; sodium 186.6mg.

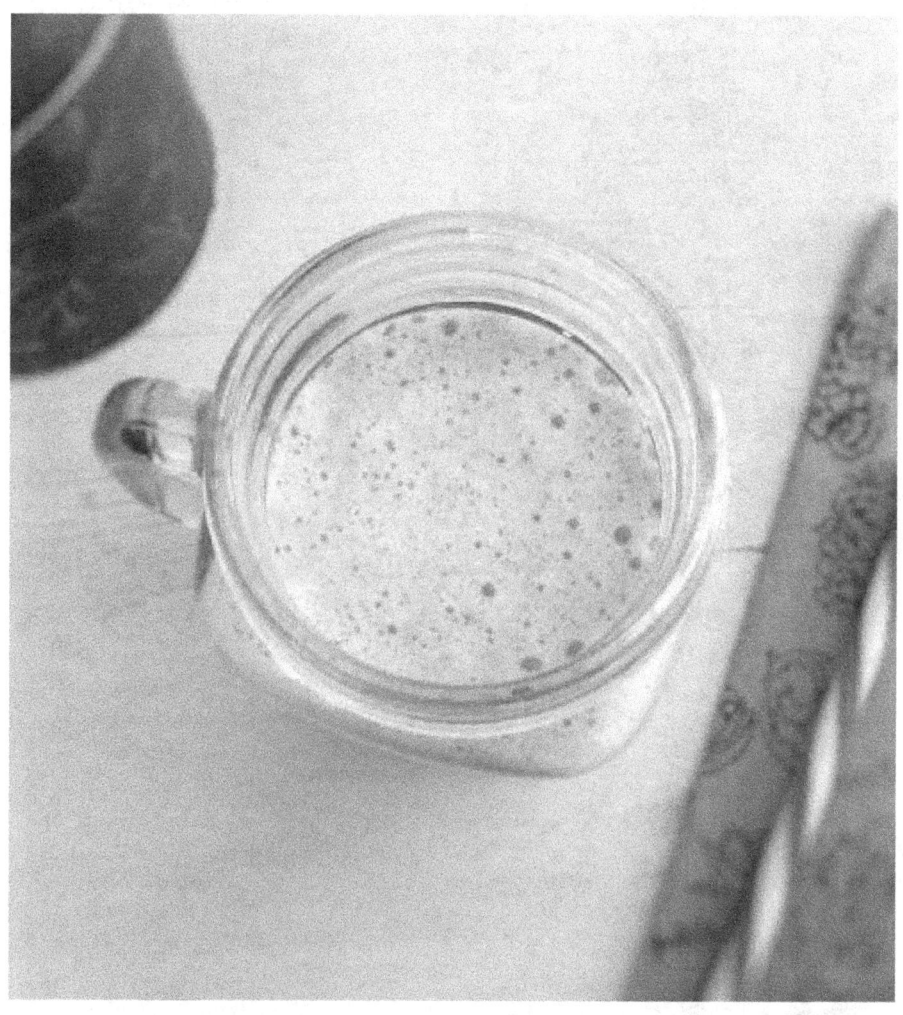

CHAPTER 6: **DESSERTS**

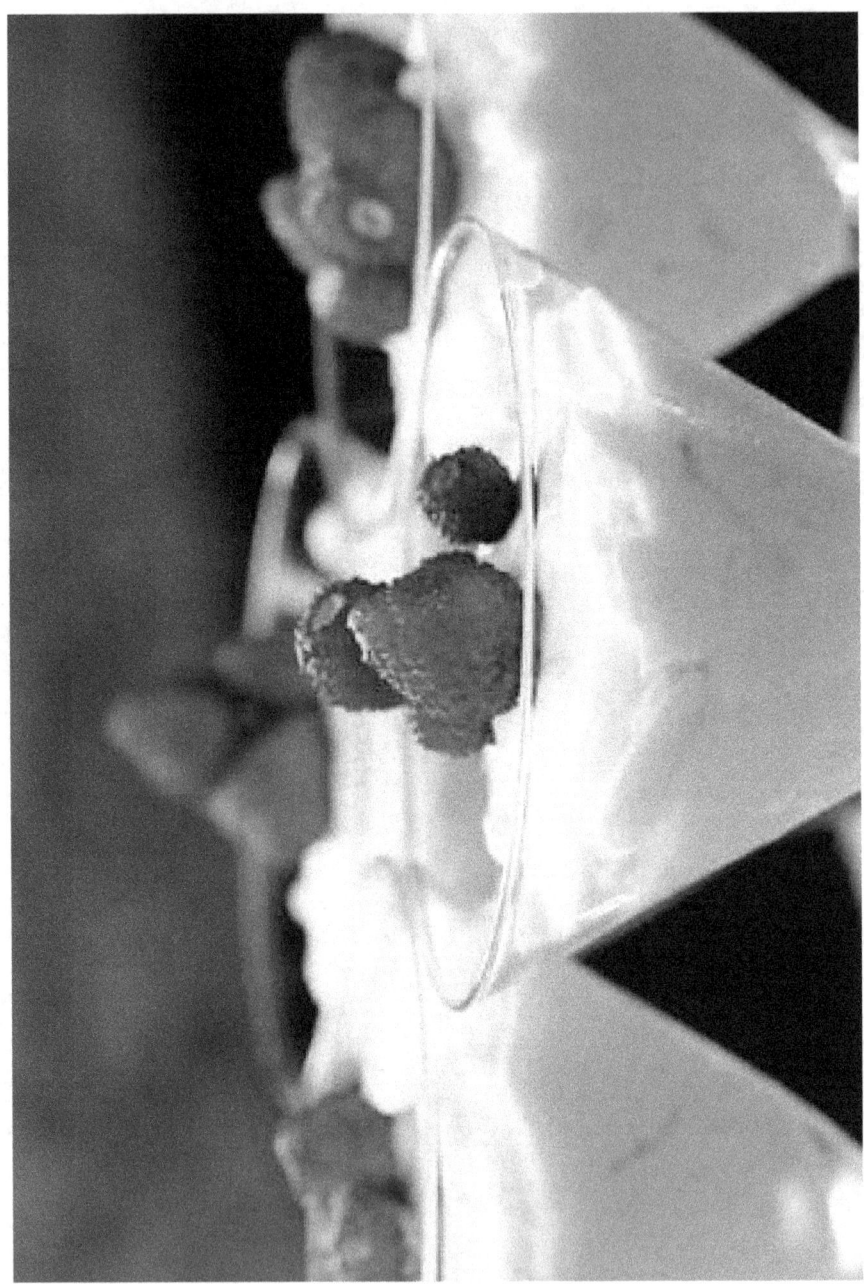

Ricotta Mousse

Prep:

10 mins

Cook:

5 mins

Total:

15 mins

Servings:

6

Yield:

6 servings

Ingredients

3 ounces unsweetened chocolate, cut into small pieces

1 teaspoon vanilla extract

⅓ cup honey

1 pound ricotta cheese

Directions

1

Place chocolate in the top of a double boiler over simmering water. Stir frequently, scraping down the sides with a rubber spatula to avoid scorching, until chocolate is melted, about 5 minutes. Allow to cool slightly.

2

Combine melted chocolate, ricotta cheese, honey, and vanilla extract in a blender; blend until smooth. Pour into dessert cups or glasses and let chill completely.

Nutrition

Per Serving: 230 calories; protein 9.4g; carbohydrates 29g; fat 9.7g; cholesterol 23.5mg; sodium 99.1mg.

Strawberry Soufflè

Prep:

40 mins

Cook:

1 hr 15 mins

Total:

1 hr 55 mins

Servings:

10

Yield:

10 servings

Ingredients

4 large egg whites egg whites, at room temperature

Pinch salt

1 cup sugar

4 cups strawberries

1 tablespoon cornstarch

1 tablespoon white vinegar

¼ teaspoon cream of tartar

1 teaspoon vanilla

2 tablespoons orange liqueur

2 cups whipping cream

Directions

1

Beat egg whites, cream of tartar and salt in a large bowl with an electric mixer until soft peaks form. Beat in sugar, 1 tbsp at a time, until stiff, glossy peaks form. Beat in cornstarch, vinegar and vanilla just until blended.

2

On a baking sheet lined with parchment paper or foil, spread meringue into a 10-inch (25 cm) circle with a raised edge and a slight indentation in the centre.

3

Bake in a preheated 250 degrees F oven until firm to the touch, about 1-1/4 hours. Meringue should be cream-coloured. If it appears to be browning, reduce oven temperature to 225 degrees F.

4

Remove from oven and let cool.

5

When ready to serve, peel parchment paper off back of meringue. Place meringue on a serving plate. Cut strawberries into halves or slices, if large. Whip cream until stiff peaks form. Gently stir in liqueur, if using. Spread whipped cream over meringue leaving edge of meringue visible. Top with strawberries. Cut into wedges to serve.

Nutrition

Per Serving: 281 calories; protein 2.8g; carbohydrates 27.9g; fat 17.8g; cholesterol 65.2mg; sodium 41.2mg.

Melon Ball

Prep:

5 mins

Total:

5 mins

Servings:

1

Yield:

1 melon ball

Ingredients

1 cup ice
1 fluid ounce melon schnapps
1 fluid ounce vodka
4 fluid ounces pineapple juice

Directions

1

Place ice, pineapple juice, schnapps, and vodka in a cocktail shaker.
Place cap on the shaker, shake, and strain into a cordial or pony glass.

Nutrition

Per Serving: 237 calories; protein 0.5g; carbohydrates 29.4g; fat 0.2g;
sodium 11.2mg.

Fruit Skewers

Prep:

20 mins

Total:

20 mins

Servings:

4

Yield:

8 skewers

Ingredients

⅛ teaspoon almond extract

⅛ teaspoon ground cinnamon

1 cup seedless grapes

½ cup vanilla Greek-style yogurt

2 tablespoons applesauce (such as Mott's® Natural Applesauce)

1 cup fresh strawberries

1 cup pineapple chunks

8 (6 inch) wooden skewers

1 cup apple chunks

Directions

1

Stir yogurt, applesauce, almond extract, and cinnamon together in a bowl until dipping sauce is well-combined.

2

Thread grapes, strawberries, apple chunks, and pineapple chunks alternatively onto skewers. Arrange finished skewers on a plate and serve with dipping sauce.

Nutrition

Per Serving: 117 calories; protein 2.5g; carbohydrates 26.2g; fat 1.3g; cholesterol 2.3mg; sodium 8.6mg.

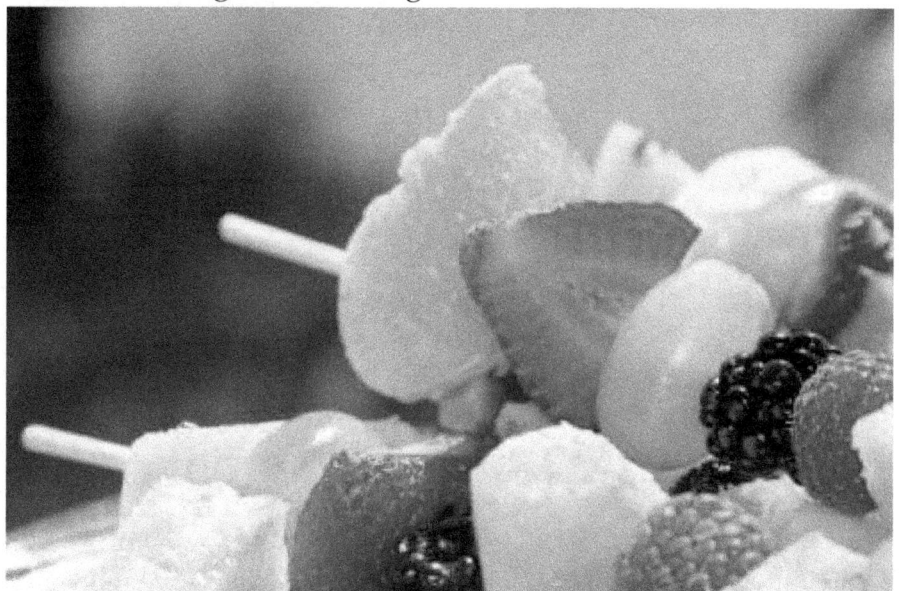

Carrot Zucchini Muffins

Prep:

25 mins

Cook:

20 mins

Total:

45 mins

Servings:

21

Yield:

21 muffins

Ingredients

1 cup butter

3 eggs

1 cup white sugar

2 cups grated zucchini

1 cup grated carrots

2 teaspoons ground cinnamon

3 teaspoons vanilla extract

3 cups all-purpose flour

2 teaspoons ground nutmeg

¼ teaspoon baking powder

1 teaspoon salt

1 teaspoon baking soda

Directions

1

Preheat the oven to 350 degrees F. Grease two 12-cup muffin tins or line cups with paper liners.

2

Combine butter, sugar, and eggs in a large bowl; beat with an electric mixer until creamy. Beat in zucchini, carrots, and vanilla extract.

3

Combine flour, nutmeg, cinnamon, salt, baking soda, and baking powder in a separate bowl. Mix into the creamed butter mixture. Stir in raisins and walnuts. Pour batter into the greased muffin cups.

4

Bake in the preheated oven until a toothpick inserted into the center comes out clean, about 18 minutes.

Nutrition

Per Serving: 227 calories; protein 3.6g; carbohydrates 28g; fat 11.6g; cholesterol 49.8mg; sodium 254.4mg.

Blueberry Granita

Prep:

15 mins

Additional:

4 hrs

Total:

4 hrs 15 mins

Servings:

4

Yield:

4 servings

Ingredients

2 ½ cups blueberries

½ cup white sugar

¾ cup water

1 tablespoon fresh lemon juice

Directions

1

Blend the blueberries and sugar in a food processor until smooth; strain through a fine-mesh strainer, pressing with a wooden spoon to separate the blueberry puree from any chunks of skin or seeds.

2

Stir the strained blueberry puree, water, and lemon juice together in a shallow glass baking dish or tray. Place the dish in the freezer; scrape and stir the blueberry mixture with a fork once an hour until evenly frozen and icy, about 4 hours. Scrape to fluff and lighten the ice crystals; spoon into chilled glasses to serve.

Nutritions

Per Serving: 149 calories; protein 0.7g; carbohydrates 38.5g; fat 0.3g; sodium 2.3mg.

Cannoli alla Siciliana

Prep:

35 mins

Cook:

10 mins

Additional:

3 hrs 45 mins

Total:

4 hrs 30 mins

Servings:

20

Yield:

20 cannoli

Ingredients

Filling:

2 pounds sheep's milk ricotta cheese

1 ½ cups confectioners' sugar

¼ cup mixed peel

1 ½ ounces dark chocolate, finely chopped

Cannoli Shells:

1 ¼ cups all-purpose flour

3 tablespoons dry Marsala wine, or more to taste

1 tablespoon butter, softened

1 tablespoon white sugar

2 teaspoons vinegar, or more to taste

corn oil for frying

Topping:

3 tablespoons chopped pistachio nuts

2 tablespoons confectioners' sugar, or to taste

Directions

1

Beat ricotta cheese and 1 1/2 cup confectioners' sugar together in a bowl until smooth. Stir in mixed peel and chocolate. Cover and refrigerate for 3 hours.

2

Mix flour, Marsala wine, butter, sugar, and vinegar together in a bowl to make cannoli dough. Wrap in plastic wrap; let rest for 30 minutes.

3

Knead dough on a lightly floured work surface until smooth. Roll to 1/8-inch thickness. Cut into twenty 4-inch squares. Wrap each square around a metal tubular mold, overlapping ends and dabbing with warm water to seal.

4

Heat oil in a large saucepan over medium-high heat. Lower some cannoli molds into the hot oil; cook until shells are golden and crisp, about 10 minutes. Drain on paper towels. Repeat with remaining cannoli molds. Cool briefly; twist molds carefully to remove shells. Let shells cool completely, about 15 minutes.

5

Fill cooled cannoli shells with ricotta filling using a spoon or piping bag. Arrange cannoli on a serving platter. Garnish with pistachios; sprinkle 2 tablespoons confectioners' sugar on top.

Nutritions

Per Serving: 177 calories; protein 6.6g; carbohydrates 25.2g; fat 5.5g; cholesterol 15.7mg; sodium 67.9mg.

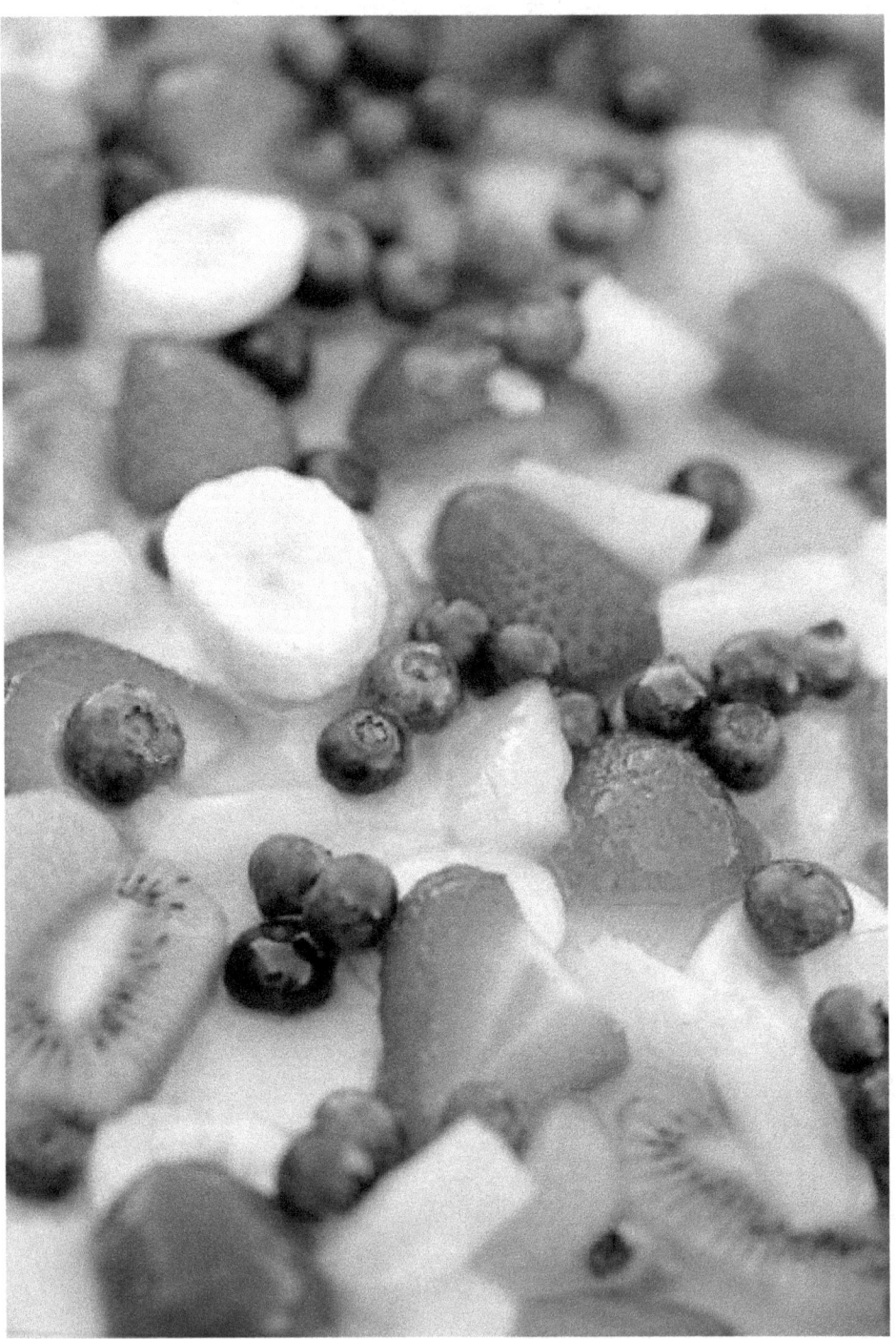

CPSIA information can be obtained
at www.ICGtesting.com
Printed in the USA
BVHW090319220621
610126BV00011B/2320